Fecal Transplant

New Treatment for Ulcerative Colitis,
Crohn's, Irritable Bowel Disease, Diarrhea,
C.diff., Multiple Sclerosis, Autism, and More.

**How to change your own gut bacteria to heal
your immune system, brain and digestive tract.**

Diane York, MS, CRC

Fecal Transplant
New Treatment for Ulcerative Colitis, Crohn's, Irritable Bowel Disease,
Diarrhea, C.diff., Multiple Sclerosis, Autism, and More.
How to change your own gut bacteria to heal your immune system, brain
and digestive tract.

ISBN: 978-0-9889734-1-1

Contents

*"The bottom line is fecal transplants work,
and not by just supplying a missing bug
but a missing function being carried out by
multiple organisms in the transplant….."*

Dr. Vincent B. Young, Associate Professor,
Department of Internal Medicine/Infectious Diseases and
the Department of Microbiology & Immunology at
the University of Michigan in Ann Arbor.

*"FMT has undergone a rapid transformation
in the past decade, from being considered an
evidence-free, alternative form of medicine
to acceptance as a mainstream treatment
option with vast therapeutic potential."*

Dr. Thomas Borody, Gastroenterologist,
Director, Centre for Digestive Diseases, Sydney, Australia

*"The experimental medical procedure known
as a Fecal Microbiota Transplant (FMT)
holds enormous therapeutic promise for both
C. difficile and a variety of other diseases."*

Brendan Pease, Fighting Infections with Feces:
The Promise of Fecal Microbiota Transplantation,
Harvard Science Review, January 22, 2014

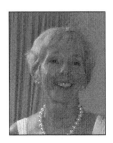

Diane York, MS, CRC

AUTHOR BIO:

A former social worker and rehabilitation counselor, Diane York is an award-winning journalist and author located in Richmond, VA. She writes extensively on health and lifestyle issues for publications in Richmond, Virginia and Sanibel, Florida.

See: *dianeyorkcreative.com.*

Why I Wrote This Book

I am a freelance writer with past careers as a social worker, rehabilitation counselor and patient evaluator in hospital brain injury programs. I know many people who have serious gastrointestinal illnesses, multiple food allergies and chemical sensitivities. Two of them are my sons. One is my granddaughter. I, myself, have had many of these same issues, as well as four long years of increasingly severe unexplained diarrhea, accompanied by nutritional deficiencies, bone loss and yeast infections. It wasn't until I found out I had gluten intolerance that things began to turn around for me health-wise. Fecal microbiota transplants have taken me to yet another level of health not enjoyed in twenty years.

I had never heard of fecal microbiota transplant until a friend became dangerously ill with ulcerative colitis, (UC.) Allie, (not her real name) had tried every drug in her doctor's playbook without much success. Desperate, she went out of the country to obtain two weeks of FMT treatment. She returned after two weeks a new woman; so improved she no longer required IV nutrition to survive.

I became even more interested when she told me that some parents were bringing their autistic children to the clinic and having good results. Not "cures" mind you. But changes, such as a child being able to return a smile when he had never smiled before, or a child beginning to talk despite years of silence. Having a granddaughter who has been diagnosed with autism made me want to know more about this therapy.

In an effort to learn as much as I could about fecal transplants, I self-administered fecal transplants at home using a thoroughly tested, very healthy friend as donor. I then traveled to the top clinic in the world, (Taymount clinic in the UK) and went through two weeks of their protocol with great results. I have read every current research paper and journal article on the topic of fecal transplant I could access.

The value of the gut microbiome to our overall health is one of the most important medical discoveries in my lifetime. Fecal transplant is a safe, easy therapy that seems to rebalance the microbiome. Testing of donor stool is critical but available to anyone who can afford the price. Most people are able to administer a transplant themselves. This treatment is saving lives in the United Kingdom, Argentina, Australia, and other countries where it is an accepted practice for many conditions. At present, in the United States, physicians are allowed to provide fecal microbiota transplants for only one medical condition, that of Clostridia difficile infection and only after several attempts using antibiotics.

It is my desire in writing this book to help others who desperately need this treatment to have all the information they need to access safe FMT or perform it themselves. It is my hope that a treatment with such potential and minimal side effects will soon become available in this country and that physicians will be permitted to utilize it for all those conditions which research has shown it can help.

CHAPTER ONE

The Basics of Fecal Transplants

Introduction to Your Gut Microbes

I f asked to identify the two key elements of good health, most people would choose diet and exercise. But there may be a third, one you might never suspect. There is growing evidence that this element is just as essential, perhaps more than the other two. It is the bacteria in your gut.

The trillions of microorganisms that live in the approximately twenty-seven feet of intestines in your body as well as in the mouth, the nose, lungs, vagina and on the skin, are called the human microbiome and some researchers consider it to be a newly discovered, critically important "organ."

All over the world, researchers in widely divergent fields of medicine are conducting studies and clinical trials on the benefits of "shit" therapy, more professionally known as fecal microbiota transplantation or FMT. That is the transplanting of bacteria extracted from fecal material from a healthy donor to a person struggling with disease. Bacteria from the microbiome may well be newest 'super drug.'

Science and medical journals are exploding with articles and clinical trials studying the role of gut bacteria and its impact on health. As of the writing of this book, there are over 509,000 online scholarly articles on the topic of gut bacteria, 331,000 on the topic of gut bacteria and the immune system, 16,500 on the topic of multiple sclerosis and gut bacteria. Even more startling is the fact that there are 76,000 articles on possible connections between gut bacteria and schizophrenia and 96,000 on gut bacteria's role in autism.

While digestive disorders are an obvious target for this treatment, now scientists are relating gut bacteria to other major systems of the body as well; the brain and the immune system. Because they now know that *ninety percent of the neurotransmitters the brain uses are made in the gut,* they are finding links to disorders including depression, bi-polar disorder and autism. In addition, they have found that *seventy percent of the immune system resides in the gut.* Thus, researchers are also looking at the possibility that gut bacteria imbalances are a cause behind the increase in auto-immune disease in this country and worldwide.

The impact of gut bacteria on general health became such a focus that in May 2016, the White House Office of Science and Technology Policy, announced a new National Microbiome Initiative (NMI) to foster the integrated study of microbiomes across different ecosystems. Just as the years 2003 to 2016 were named the Era of the Human Genome (study of the human gene), President Obama named this the Era of the Human Microbiome.

Within the past decade, two large projects were funded that also reflect the importance of the human microbiome. The Human Microbiome Project (HMP) is a United States National Institutes of Health (NIH) initiative created in 2008 to identify and study how changes in the microorganisms within our bodies affect human health and disease.

And, professor Rob Knight, Ph.D. of the University of California-San Diego, co-founded the huge American Gut Project in 2012. This is an ongoing endeavor to create a "library" of thousands of fecal samples from volunteers all across the country. As of November 11, 2013, it had collected over 2,000 samples from volunteers. The data from these studies is being used for research over a wide field of medical conditions including irritable bowel syndrome, celiac disease, multiple sclerosis, Parkinson's disease, autism, mood disorders and other conditions affecting the central nervous system.

All of this information and research is creating a paradigm shift in understanding how the systems in the human body function and interact.

ALLIE'S STORY

Allie, at age thirty-seven, was tall, with elegant features and a positive, outgoing personality. She had a successful career as a high-energy real estate saleswoman. She was going strong except for one thing, she was suffering with ulcerative colitis (UC.) Ulcerative colitis is an autoimmune disease in which the body attacks its own tissues destroying the lining of the large intestines or colon, producing inflammation and ulcerations. As a result, the digestive tract loses its ability to get nutrition from the food we eat. Effects are unpredictable episodes of diarrhea, abdominal pain, loss of weight, fatigue, anemia and weakness. Allie was trying to control it with doctor's visits, prednisone, a special diet, and other medications but her symptoms continued to worsen. Working was getting difficult due to the bouts of diarrhea and fatigue from loss of nutrition.

Her disease was causing Allie to lose a half-pound per week. As her weight plummeted from 145 to 100 pounds, her iron levels dropped too. A normal iron level for a woman is between twelve to fifteen.[1] Her level was a frightening three.

With less iron to transport oxygen through her body, her heart was pumping harder to compensate, putting this once-vibrant young woman at risk of heart failure. She tried all the current medications for her condition without success. As her health and her life spiraled out of control, Allie had to stop working. Allie's doctor prescribed intravenous nutrition to stabilize her weight and scheduled blood transfusions to boost her iron levels. But these measures provided only temporary relief. Her only option, her doctor said, would come from removing her colon. The surgery would leave Allie with a colostomy bag for the rest of her life.

But Allie had learned about a new therapy called fecal microbiota transplant or FMT. As mentioned previously, fecal transplants are the transfer of bacteria from donated excrement that has been screened for disease and pathogens to another person. This can be done via an enema, endoscopy, colonoscopy or in some cases a pill made from dried fecal material. The goal is to replenish the gut with healthy bacteria.

FMT is a relatively unknown therapy in the United States. Here, it is FDA approved only for cases of Clostridium difficile, a nasty, drug-resistant intestinal infection that kills thousands in the US each year. But there are clinics in Great Britain, Australia, the Bahamas and other countries that have been utilizing FMT for years to treat a variety of gastric problems. The cost could be anywhere from $5,000 to $10,000, plus travel expenses. Allie was tight on money. Her parents and grandparents were deceased. She was on her own and had been out of work long enough to use most of her savings, but she was desperate.

Physically weak, she did not think she could handle the plane ride to Great Britain. She chose the clinic in the Bahamas, a much closer travel destination. She enlisted a friend to go with her. Just getting a passport and making travel arrangements were difficult in her weakened condition. The trip would be a challenge considering her diarrhea problem and food sensitivities which made eating at restaurants almost impossible. And, she'd be forced to abandon the intravenous nutrition that had stabilized her weight. Still, she needed relief and hoped to avoid a surgery that would leave her physically compromised for life, so she went.

Half-way through her first week of treatment, she was amazed to find that her diarrhea and colitis spasms were reduced. They were still a problem but so much less so, she was excited and hopeful. For the first time in years, she was able to go to the beach and sit in the sun, and she began to believe she might have a real life again.

"Halfway through my first week at the clinic, having received treatments for three days, I felt a big difference. For one thing, my bowel movements, which had been about ten a day, were reduced to about five. This was a huge difference for me. But also, I felt it had affected my immune system, I felt stronger, more in control and definitely more optimistic," Allie explained.

She came home a week later. She would continue with several more treatments (self-administered via enema) at home. She was a different person, a stronger voice, hopeful and positive. She still has a long way to go, her diarrhea, while reduced, is still a huge problem and the number and kinds of food she can eat are limited, but she is on the upswing and feels she finally has seen some improvement in her health. (Note: Clinical studies of FMT for colitis and Crohn's are finding that a six to eight-week trial rather than a two-week trial has brought about remission lasting a year or more in patients that participated.)

Is This You?

So, the medicine that improved Allie's condition was ten doses of gut bacteria from other people. Who would have guessed?

You, or someone you love, may experience random bouts of diarrhea, stomach pains after eating, unrelenting acid reflux, constipation, abdominal pains, embarrassing gas and belching, allergies, reactions to foods, cramps, fatigue, depression, anxiety and/or insomnia. One or more of these symptoms may be driving you crazy. Your doctor may run the traditional tests and can't find a thing, making you feel like a hypochondriac.

If so, you may be one of the thousands of people in the US who have some variation of inflammatory bowel disease. According to the National Institutes of Health, gastrointestinal diseases affect between 60 and 70 million Americans each year. These include: ulcerative colitis, celiac disease, Crohn's Disease, irritable bowel syndrome, diverticulitis, diverticulosis, gluten intolerance, soy intolerance, casein (milk protein) intolerance and many others.

Digestive problems may seem mild, in fact, you may not even know you have a problem or they can be so severe that they control your life. But, even if you are not aware that you have a problem, the long-term effects of digestive issues may be serious or even life-threatening. Some of the side effects of these hard to diagnose digestive problems may be malnutrition, anemia, osteoporosis, dangerously low iron levels, fatigue and depression. They may also be involved in causing autoimmune diseases.

Clinics and private physicians who perform FMT for patients with Clostridia difficile (C.diff) infections have published case studies that show that, in some cases, in addition to curing the C.diff infection, remission of autoimmune disease symptoms resulted. Clinical studies are being conducted with patients who have various autoimmune diseases to see if these results can be replicated. (See the chapter in this book on autoimmune disease.)

The Role of Gut Bacteria in Human Health

How does all this happen? The average human body has about 40 trillion cells of bacteria and about 30 trillion human cells. The bacteria in our bodies actually outweighs the human cells. Much of it is located in our small and large intestines. Usually the relationship between us and that bacteria is a friendly one, with both parties enjoying mutual benefits. The bacteria work hard for their upkeep, helping turn food into fuel for the body, helping to regulate the immune system and keeping bad bugs from harming us. Some kinds of bacteria are essential in small doses, but in large doses, they can be lethal. That delicate balance is everything. It is said that each person's bacterial makeup is similar to a fingerprint, being specific to that individual. And the makeup and balance of that bacteria can determine our whole-body health. Our gut bacteria package is affected by things such as whether we were born by C-section, whether we were breast fed, the food we eat, antibiotics we take as medication and antibiotics in our food chain, where we live and the quality of our air and water.

An April 2015 article in the *Journal of Molecular Science* summarizes the impact of gut bacteria on human health. Based on substantiated clinical reports and trials, the authors state: "Gut bacteria have been found to be involved in many diseases, such as inflammatory bowel disease, obesity, diabetes, carcinoma, HIV, and autism. Immuno-regulatory activity is the main function of gut bacteria in the pathogenesis of these diseases. In recent years, prebiotics and probiotics have been widely used in the treatment of some diseases and have shown great effects. Fecal microbiota transplant is also a way to modulate gut bacteria."[2]

History of Fecal Transplants

As you might suspect, the history of fecal transplants is an unusual one. FMT is, comparatively speaking, a very new therapy in the Western world. But it was used by the Chinese as far back as the fourth century as a treatment for food poisoning and diarrhea. It was called "yellow soup," a mixture of fermented human stool and water, which was consumed by the patient. Yumm! And in Egypt, the Ebers Papyrus, a document from ancient Egypt dating back to 1500 BC, contains more than fifty prescriptions for medicines that incorporate human feces as the active ingredient. In the 17th century, an Italian anatomist named Fabricius ab Aquapendente was using stool to treat gastrointestinal diseases in veterinary medicine. There are also references to the use of fresh camel feces (eaten) by the Bedouins as a remedy for dysentery. German soldiers stationed in Africa during World War II attested to its efficacy.

Here, in the United States, the first articles published in medical journals on this topic came about in the early 1950s. The report that got the most widespread attention came in 1958, when Chief of Surgery at Denver General Hospital, Dr. Ben Eiseman, reported in the *Journal of Clinical Gastroenterology*, a story of four patients who were cured of pseudomembraneous colitis, also now known as C.diff. Enemas containing feces from healthy colons successfully replenished good digestive bacteria in these patients.[3]

But, the first widely publicized contemporary uses of fecal transplants to cure human disease began with doctors who were willing to risk ridicule to try new therapies to save dying patients.

In the mid-1980s, Australian gastroenterologist, Professor Thomas Borody, (of the Centre for Digestive Diseases in Sydney, Australia) who invented the triple antibiotic therapy for helicobacter pylori bacterium (H. pylori) (the cause of stomach ulcers), was faced with one of the most difficult cases he had seen at that time. His patient was a woman who had developed an incurable colitis through an unidentifiable pathogen after vacationing on the island of Fiji. He searched medical literature for alternative treatments and came across the paper which was published in 1958 by Dr. Eiseman. Dr. Borody used this paper as a basis for his own FMT procedure.

BABY POOP?

Where do you think all those probiotics in your yogurt come from?

Well, the first strains of Lactobacillus rhamnosus GG, found in a variety of yogurts and daily dose drinks, were isolated from human feces in 1983. In Spain, they have been experimenting using probiotics to ferment sausages. The bacteria they use is sourced from the fecal material of healthy babies up to six months old.

Ref: Jofre, Anna, Rubio, R, et al, Nutritionally enhanced fermented sausages as a vehicle for potential probiotic lactobacilli delivery, *Meat Science*, Vol. 96, Volume 96, Issue 2, Part A, February 2014, Pages 937-942.

The woman's brother donated stool which was screened for known pathogens. Using a blender, Professor Borody mixed saline with the stool and made a slush which he filtered to remove any solids. He administered it to his patient by enema on two consecutive days. The results were incredible, and her colitis was gone within days and never returned.

The cure rate for C. diff, according to Professor Borody is around 95% after the first transplant and close to 100% for the second. His clinic in Sydney, Australia is one of the top centers in the world for FMT treatment. He has used fecal transplant extensively since the 1980s and has published over 135 articles on the topic.

In the decades since Dr. Eiseman's revolutionary treatment and publication of its results, the rate of C. diff exploded and fecal transplants or FMTs, suddenly became an important medical story. Between 2012 and 2013, as numerous reports were released from medical researchers, articles began appearing in popular national publications. *Scientific*

America, National Geographic, a series of articles in *Wired,* among others, all presented stories of how successful FMT was for C.diff and other digestive disorders. In December of 2011, *Wired* author Maryn McKenna said: "Fecal transplants that cure intestinal diseases are minimally invasive, reliable, cheap and have a durable clinical history."

In 2013, an article was published in the New England Journal of Medicine reporting on a clinical trial using FMT on a group of patients who had resistant Clostridium difficile. That article was widely read and provided proof that FMT was effective in curing C. diff. FMT gained immediate credibility.[4]

At that time, FMT also began to be used in the United States for colitis sufferers. It was inexpensive, easy, involved little danger to the patient and had an extremely high success rate as therapies go.

As it became more widely used, the FDA suddenly moved in May 2013, to classify fecal microbiota transplant as both an investigational new drug (IND) and a biologic (a drug made from living organisms). They set in place a regulation that allowed only physicians currently in possession of an approved investigational new drug application to continue performing fecal transplant.

As a result, almost overnight, only twenty physicians in the US could legally perform this procedure. An outcry from the public and the medical community moved the FDA, six weeks later, to reverse their decision and allow qualified physicians to perform FMT but only for cases of recurrent C. diff where antibiotics had failed three times, and only with signed consents from patients, using donor stool that had been tested.

This was a serious restriction. It made this cheap, safe treatment unavailable to thousands of individuals with digestive disorders that can ultimately be life-threating. I recently called the FDA and asked what it would take for the FDA to reconsider its position on FMT. I was told it would require a strong lobbying effect on the part of physicians and citizens to open another hearing on the topic.

In many other countries, (Great Britain, the Bahamas and Australia, among others) FMT is an accepted treatment for other conditions such as constipation, chronic diarrhea, chronic fatigue syndrome, Crohn's Disease, ulcerative colitis, dysbiosis, irritable bowel syndrome and leaky gut. There have been reports too of amelioration of symptoms of multiple sclerosis, Parkinson's Disease and autism, even when the treatment was intended for a digestive problem. While it is available overseas, it is expensive. In addition to the travel cost, charges for two weeks of the procedure run from $5,000 to $10,000.

Because of this, many individuals have turned to finding and testing their own donors and doing FMT themselves at home.

The C.diff. Epidemic and FMT

In his book, *Tragedy, Shit and How I Saved the World,* (2016) Dave Stebbins describes a fictional scenario in which a serious bacterial infection spreads across the globe, creating an apocalyptic world in which much of the population is dying. His character tries to figure out what is wrong and sees that certain people seem immune to this contagion. He talks a Latino housekeeper, who is healthy, into giving him some of her excrement and then creates an enema with the material, with which he saves his neighbor, himself and ultimately thousands of others. Think this is ridiculous? Maybe not.

Clostridium difficile (C. diff) could well be the infection Dave Stebbins was talking about in his novel. Widespread use of antibiotics has helped to create drug resistant strains of this bacteria. C.diff is a mean bug that tears up the gut, producing uncontrolled diarrhea and bleeding. It kills Americans at the rate of 15,000 a year. Most of the infections begin in hospital or nursing home settings where they spread quickly among immune challenged patients. If your gut bacteria are already weakened by antibiotics or any other cause, you are fair game. As mentioned above, doctors found that the cure rate, using FMT was 95 % after one application. While the rate of cure using antibiotics such as Vancomycin is similar, (97%), about 25% of patients develop a resistant strain following antibiotic treatment, (thus increasing the risk of death). With FMT there is greatly reduced chance of development of an antibiotic resistant strain if the patient is treated with FMT alone. For patients who develop antibiotic resistant C. diff., fecal transplant is the only alternative.

C. diff caused almost half a million infections among patients in the United States in a single year, according to a study released by the Centers for Disease Control and Prevention (CDC) in 2015. Approximately 29,000 patients died within 30 days of the initial diagnosis of C. difficile. Of those, about 15,000 deaths were estimated to be directly attributable to C. difficile infections.[5]

C. diff. is caused by an overgrowth of the bacteria Clostridia diffi-cile. C. diff infections usually occur when someone is exposed to the pathogen while receiving antibiotic treatment for some other illness. Antibiotics suppress the normal bacteria in the colon, allowing C. diff to flourish, producing toxins that cause severe diarrhea. Damage to the colon can cause bacteria to leak into the bloodstream. Symptoms include watery diarrhea and abdominal pain over several days. Severe cases would include fever and blood or pus in the stool and uncon-trolled diarrhea. *Today, astoundingly, one of every nine patients over the age of 65, dies within 30 days of diagnosis*, according to the CDC., a truly frightening statistic.

Where We are Today

The regulations that made it illegal for physicians to perform FMT for any condition other than C. diff may have put many people at high risk from serious diseases such as colitis and Crohn's disease and other conditions that have been shown to be helped by FMT therapy. This has created an underground movement in which people are taking the treatment into their own hands, finding and testing donors and creating their own FMT implants. People desperate for treatment may take shortcuts in testing and handling stool that may lead to disaster. All of which could be avoided by having this treatment available through your own gastrointestinal physician.

THE CATHERINE DUFF STORY

In 2013, Catherine Duff, dying from antibiotic resistant C.diff, was ready to give up. She had endured eight bouts of C.diff infections. She lay in bed for months, in pain, with constant diarrhea, not knowing if she would live another day. She would recover temporarily after receiving antibiotics, but the infection came back, seemingly worse each time. Her physicians said there was nothing more they could do. She and her husband were desperate. An answer came, not from her doctors but from her daughter, who had done research online and found information about the success of FMT with C. diff cases. They did more research, had her husband's stool tested and performed an in-home enema. Within twenty-four hours, all of the symptoms of her disease were gone. The family was astonished and overjoyed. Her full story and personal plea to the FDA to legalize the use of FMT by physicians in the US can be seen at the conclusion of this book.

Why is my GI Doctor Not Talking to Me about Gut Bacteria?

In the 1980's Barry Marshall, an Australian doctor made the claim, based on his research, that (H. Pylori) bacteria was the cause of peptic ulcers. He was ridiculed by the medical establishment, which still told patients their ulcers were caused by stress. However, twenty years later, he was awarded the Nobel Prize for that discovery. This is not unusual. Science, in general, takes time to be accepted by both the scientific community and the people who benefit from it. This is especially true when there are ingrained belief systems that contradict the new information.

With the invention of the internet, however, innovative ideas can spread much faster and be studied by researchers all over the world, helping to break down barriers of thought that may predominate in one country.

The FDA regulations on FMT as an "investigational drug" will considerably slow down research in the United States that could prove its value for conditions other than C. diff.

While many universities and non-profits are attempting to aggressively research FMT's therapeutic benefits, there is very little funding for the study of this treatment. That may be because there are limited ways to make money from its use. You can't patent bacteria that already exists in fecal microbiota. Glenn Taylor, Director of the Taymount Clinic in England, says: "the major pharmaceutical companies would not want a relatively cheap and effective solution to be used to replace expensive and on-going pharmacological drugs and they will not be in favor of doctors trying anything so natural and freely available as feces to bring about the drug-free remission called health."

Vancocin, an oral form of the antibiotic Vancomycin, the drug of choice for C.diff, sold by ViroPharma, costs $1,000 to $1,500 for a 10- to 14-day course of treatment at the lowest dose. Some patients get higher doses or longer treatments, multiplying the cost. Humira, only one of the many drugs prescribed for Crohn's disease and colitis, generates over ten billion dollars annually for its manufacturer, Abbott Labs. Unlike fecal transplant which has no side effects, Humira works by tamping down the immune system, leaving you vulnerable to infections, viruses and pathogens. The warning label says: *"Serious infections have happened in people taking HUMIRA. These serious infections include tuberculosis (TB) and infections caused by viruses, fungi, or bacteria that have spread throughout the body."*

Taylor adds that other reasons for the lack of acceptance of fecal transplant may be: "In reading mainstream articles written by physicians, we have found repeated reference to the "Yuk" factor. It might just be that doctors just don't want to get involved with something as basic as feces. Doctors, during their extensive medical training, do not get enough training in the basic biological and microbiological world of gut microbes and what feces really contain." He adds that as long as we wait for "the drug companies to come up with a pill for every ill, the doctors will continue to study medicine and not biology."

When we look at both the amount of research and the availability of FMT as a treatment in other countries, as opposed to our severe constraints on its use in this country, it may be that we are missing out on one of the most promising therapies for a wide spectrum of conditions. The research studies, clinical trials and case studies are exciting and promising for a variety of medical conditions.

The Promise of Research

At the time of this writing, there are over 100 clinical trials dealing with FMT listed on the United States government clinical trials website. This does not include the numerous trials being conducted in other countries. Most of these trials are for treating the infection known as C. diff. However, there are also trials for conditions such as: Parkinson's disease, Crohn's disease, colitis, obesity, IBS, diabetes, liver transplant, cirrhosis of the liver, autism and metabolic syndrome. (Metabolic syndrome is the name for a group of risk factors that raises your risk for heart disease and other health problems, such as diabetes and stroke.)

In his 2013 article in the *Current Gastrointestinal Reports*, Thomas Borody, one of the world's foremost researchers on the use of FMT, said: "FMT has undergone a rapid transformation in the past decade, from being considered an evidence-free, alternative form of medicine to acceptance as a mainstream treatment option with vast therapeutic potential."[6]

That perspective was affirmed in an article in the January 2015 issue of the *World Journal of Gastroenterology*. The article, "Fecal microbiota transplantation broadening its application beyond intestinal disorders" is a review of current journal articles on the topic of FMT and explains that intestinal dysbiosis (overgrowth of fungal or bacteria in the intestines) is now known to be a complication in many different disease processes.

It goes on to point out that while fecal microbiota transplantation, is being used effectively for curing the Clostridium difficile infection, there is substantial evidence it may also be useful in the management of other disorders including metabolic diseases, neuropsychiatric disorders, autoimmune diseases and allergic disorders. An unexpected byproduct of FMT can be a difference in tendency to gain or lose weight and changes in insulin resistance in the person receiving the implant. "Case reports of FMT have also shown favorable outcomes in Parkinson's disease, multiple sclerosis, myoclonus dystonia, chronic fatigue syndrome, and idiopathic thrombocytopenic purpura."[7]

No one can pretend to know the complete life cycle or all the varieties of even a single species of bacteria. It would be an assumption to think so.

Ernst Almquist,
a colleague of Dr. Louis Pasteur.

CHAPTER TWO

Fantastic Beasts and Where to Find Them

Amazing Bacteria

Here are some riddles: What creature can stay alive for 34,000 years? What organism can be resurrected after forty million years? What is it that can survive boiling water and live in below-freezing temperatures? What can steal genes from other life forms and transform itself?

While our human ancestors evolved about six million years ago, something else had a big head start. Bacteria have been here for three billion years and are an incredibly diverse and talented life form. Some bacteria can steal genes from other bacteria and then develop new skills. Can you imagine being able to fly by eating a bird? Or learning to breathe under water by holding a fish? The process is called horizontal gene transfer, an amazing ability to change your own DNA.

Bacteria have been found living in frozen glaciers and in hot springs with temperatures of 252 degrees Fahrenheit. Called extremophiles, they are the newest stars of the bacteria world. Their ability to survive temperature variations make life on hostile planets seem plausible. In the boiling water of Yellowstone's hot springs, strange forms of bacteria learned to defend themselves from viruses by cutting up their adversaries' DNA. The process is called CRISPR (clustered regularly interspaced short palindromic repeats.) Scientists are now using CRISPR to edit sequences of DNA giving them the ability to easily make genetic changes in organisms. Applications of this are mind blowing.[8,9,10]

The tiny purple microbe, called Herminiimonas glaciei, was found under two miles of ice in Greenland. Scientists estimate it was trapped there over 120,000 years ago. It was revived over an eleven-month period by gradual warming in an incubator. Finally, it was alive again and actively reproducing new colonies of bacteria.[11]

Some bacteria know how to produce light (bioluminescence) and scientists have developed a special kind of bacteria that actually begins to glow in the presence of landmines. When proteins on the surface of E. coli detect TNT, this turns on the gene responsible for light production. This discovery could revolutionize locating landmines lying in wait in eighty-seven countries of the world.[12]

Some microbes can eat oil and some collect radioactive materials from the soil. Both could provide ways to clean up hazardous materials. Bacteria, and other microbes such as microalgae and fungi, are now being used in a wide variety of technologies. Patent fights are numerous over these unique forms of life. Biotechnology is finding applications for bacteria in materials processing, energy production, waste processing and bioremediation, corrosion resistance, production of drugs and the manufacture of polymers.

The array of talents and skills in bacteria, their resilience and variety make the study of microbiology and bacteriology an incredible Pandora's Box of surprises, gifts and dangers.

It's Alive!

Showering each day, shampooing your hair and washing your hands with sanitizers may make you feel like you are clean. But you're not. Your body is covered with squirming, wriggling microscopic creatures. They are in your mouth, your nose, your genitals, your armpits, under your breasts, between your legs, down your throat, and especially in your stomach, your guts and out your anus and in your vagina. You can't wash them all off or wash them all out. They will be on you and in you every day until you die. All of this may sound yucky, but these critters are vitally important.

Some are your deadly enemies; just waiting to get a foothold in your body so they can overwhelm you. Yet others are your very best friends. Without them, you can't digest food, think a clear thought, or pass waste material from your body.

While the number of bacterial cells in the body is close to the number of human cells, the variety of bacterial cells is astounding. We have about 200 types of human cells but ten thousand species of bacteria have been identified in and on the human body and that may be just a drop in the bacterial bucket.[13]

Our gut microbes, by themselves, can weigh about three pounds. One third of our gut bacteria is similar in most people, while two thirds are specific to each one of us. The composition of species is highly personalized and usually determined by our environment and our diet. It can adapt over time in different ethnic groups to digest specific foods commonly found in their environment. For example, people of Japanese ancestry can digest seaweeds because their microbiota has acquired special enzymes from centuries of eating seaweed.

History of Bacteria

Despite the fact that these creatures have such an integral role in our lives, causing both health and disease, we had no awareness of their existence until relatively recent times. In the 1660's a Dutch cloth merchant, Anton van Leeuwenhoek, became an expert at grinding magnifying lenses so he could examine the weave of cloth more easily. He was able to achieve magnifications up to 500 times the actual life size.

Out of curiosity, he used one of his lenses to examine a few drops of pond water. When he did, he saw that it was swarming with tiny living creatures. Leeuwenhoek sent a report of his sightings of bacteria and algae to the Royal Society in London with illustrations. His highly detailed drawings are still in existence and show a wide variety of algae and other single-celled plants and animals. From his discoveries, scientists knew that the world teemed with small organisms. However, it took two hundred years for us to figure out that bacteria could be a factor in causing some of the diseases that passed from one person to another.

The next jump in bacteria awareness occurred in the 1840's when a doctor in Vienna, Ignaz Semmelweis, working in a maternity ward realized that a ward run by midwives had a much higher survival rate for mothers and babies than did the maternity ward run by physicians. The deaths were caused by "childbed fever" or puerperal fever but no one knew the cause. Semmelweis realized that the midwives washed their hands between patients and kept the birthing areas clean. The doctors did not. They were spreading the bacteria from patient to patient. Semmelweis suggestion that doctors clean up between patients and wear clean coats for the ward and different clothing for the room where post mortems were carried out as an experiment achieved a huge drop in death rates. It also earned him many enemies. His pointing out that the midwives did a better job than the physicians resulted in his colleagues getting him fired from his position.

Proof of the bacteria-disease connection came from Louis Pasteur and Robert Koch in the 1870's. Pasteur showed that microorganisms grew in broth in a sealed tube, but no growth or spoiling of the broth occurred if it was boiled first. Boiling killed the bacteria and other microorganisms and the process or boiling to keep food fresh is still called pasteurization.

The relevance of bacteria to our health is just beginning to be studied and considering the vast numbers of bacteria and its amazing breadth of effects, skills and abilities it may be generations before we become fully aware of its possibilities as a cause and cure of disease.

How We Acquire Bacteria

We are not born with a full set of bacteria. In particular, babies are born with a "sterile" gut. Important bacteria are gained as the baby passes through the mother's birth canal, from her skin contact, and from prebiotics (that provide nourishment for microbes) in mother's breastmilk. So, it is not just genes that are passed down from generation to generation but also bacteria. The implications of this are significant as diseases previously thought to be genetic in cause, (because they were seen multiple times in the same family,) might actually be caused by bacteria passed down from the mother. Or, the lack of a certain bacteria in a family over generations could cause a disease to appear repeatedly in the same family.

So, children who are delivered by C Section or who were not breastfed are missing some of these early bacteria. The rest comes from exposures the baby has to people and things and the food and drink it consumes. The full microbiome takes from birth to about age three to completely develop. It generally remains stable through life, (unless health-related events such as illness or antibiotic use affect it) but will diminish in quantity and variety as we age.

Besides food and drink, we take in bacteria from our environment through our noses, mouths, vagina, anus, lungs, pores and/or cuts in our skin. When we touch, when we inhale, when we have sex, we are exchanging and collecting bacteria.

Because of the wide role gut microbiota plays in the working of the body and the different functions it accomplishes, experts nowadays consider it as an acquired "organ" critical to good health, an organ that needs looking after.

How Bacteria Works to Help the Body

When we eat, we chew our food, add saliva to it and swallow. Then the stomach acids and enzymes take over, breaking down the food into a manageable soft mass. But the important part occurs when the food material passes into the intestines. There's a reason the intestines are so long, winding around and around like a long string of coiled sausages. All those feet of intestine, filled with various bacteria and enzymes serve to break the food down further, giving the body the maximum opportunity to pull nutrition out of it. The "sausage links" are connected by junctures. The food should pass slowly and consistently through these junctures. All along this path to the colon, the gut bacteria does its thing; absorbing fats, vitamins, nutrients, carbs and bacteria from food and magically transforming it all into energy, hormones, neurotransmitters and creating various vitamins including Vitamin D and Vitamin K.

Fermentation is another job that bacteria perform in the body. Fermentation is a process that converts sugar to acids, gases or alcohol. While yeasts are used to ferment wine and beer, bacteria ferments nutrients to produce short-chain fatty acids, along with gases such as hydrogen, methane and carbon dioxide. The short-chain fatty acids are mostly used as an energy source, and the gases are removed in the breath or as flatulence. It has been estimated that up to ten percent of the energy our body uses comes from this fermentation process.

But the two most significant functions the microbiome performs are relatively recent discoveries. The gut produces ninety percent of the neurotransmitters our brain uses and seventy percent of our immune system is maintained by our gut bacteria. Those little bugs are responsible for a lot more than digestion.

CHAPTER THREE

Safety of Fecal Microbiota Transplants

Safety of FMT

When compared to many medical procedures (and to the side effects of major pharmaceuticals used for conditions like Crohn's and Colitis,) FMT has minimal side effects and is considered a very low risk procedure. If proper procedure is followed, FMT can be performed by anyone capable of giving themselves an enema. In fact, the simpler you keep this procedure the less risk there is, with one caveat. That is, that the donor must be *tested rigorously*. Common side effects reported include abdominal discomfort, bloating, flatulence, diarrhea, constipation and rarely, transient fever.

It is important to note that serious adverse effects, while rare, tend to occur as a result of the delivery method not from the microbiota material itself.

The Four Ways to Introduce Fecal Microbiota

There are four methods of introducing fecal microbiota transplants.

Fecal microbiota can be delivered via <u>colonoscopy.</u> Using this method entails the typical risks of colonoscopy, including damage or penetration of the colon wall as well as the risks of sedation.

It can be introduced via <u>endoscopy</u> with nasogastric tubes. In this case the tube goes all the way through the nose and down through the stomach and into the small intestine. There can be injury from the insertion or removal of the tube. This can also lead to accidental distribution of the fecal material into the stomach, leading to regurgitation of fecal material and possible aspiration of material into the lungs.

There are also <u>capsules</u> with fecal matter inside that can be swallowed. Again, in this case, there is a risk that the capsule might open in the stomach, not in the intestine. Or, if a person has difficulty swallowing they could regurgitate an opened capsule again, inducing risk of aspiration. This "top-down" method can result in small intestinal bacterial overgrowth (SIBO) if the capsule breaks before reaching the colon as the small (upper) intestine is designed to harbor few bacteria, while a healthy large intestine and colon should be rich with multiple kinds of bacteria. While in the future capsules may be fool-proof, at present, it is safest if oral delivery is performed only by a professional in a medical setting.

The easiest and safest method of delivery, in my opinion, is through <u>enema</u> into the rectum. Here, the bacteria is placed right where it is supposed to end up (no pun intended.) In clinics, it is usually delivered this way, with no more than a six-inch long insertion tube. Individuals doing this at home usually use empty, plastic, disposable enema bottles that have no more than a three-inch nozzle. They can also use the old-fashioned rubber enema bags and tubing with a nozzle about two inches long.

At a conference in Amsterdam in 2016, descriptions of what can go wrong with nasogastric implant of fecal material were abundant in a study presented.

Dr. Yvette van Beurden, at the European Society of Clinical Microbiology and Infectious Diseases Annual Congress in April 2016, shared a study of thirty-nine C.diff patients, all of whom underwent FMT. Nasogastric implant was the method of delivery for all. The study had a high clinical cure rate of 97%. However, four of the thirty-nine had adverse side effects of regurgitation of fecal material requiring immediate medical attention and hospitalization. One died from pneumonia following aspiration of material. Dr. van Beurden said this method of transplant was used because it required no anesthesia and because all the patients had inflamed colons. However, most of the patients successfully treated in clinics with enema style implantation also have inflamed colons from digestive disease.[14]

Additionally, Wang, et al, in a review of adverse effects (AE) following FMT, commented: "Route of fecal infusion is another concern in FMT that may lead to AEs. Lower gastrointestinal routes, including colonoscopy, sigmoidoscopy, and retention enema, were more widely used than upper gastrointestinal routes. We found that the patients who received FMT treatment via upper gastrointestinal routes were more likely to develop adverse effects than those who received FMT treatment via lower gastrointestinal routes (43.9% vs. 20.6%). To avoid injury associated adverse effects during endoscopic process, noninvasive and patient-acceptable routes can be chosen for FMT treatment."[15]

Most studies of FMT involve individuals who already have a serious pre-existing condition such as ulcerative colitis, Clostridia difficile infections or Crohn's Disease. In published reports of adverse effects following FMT most could be attributed to a pre-existing or pre-disposing condition so cause could not be directly connected with the FMT treatment.

Potential Long-term Adverse Events

A greater concern with FMT is the long-term. It is a relatively new therapy without years of follow up with large pools of patients. Such risks include the possible transmission of infectious agents via FMT or development of diseases/conditions related to changes in the gut microbiota. There is the theoretical possibility of transmission of unrecognized infectious agents that cause illness years after contact, similar to experiences with hepatitis C and human immunodeficiency virus. However, it is reasonable to assume that such agents would induce disease in donors as well and be picked up during donor testing. So, the best clinics and stool banks freeze and quarantine stool for about three months after donation to follow the health of the donor in case he, while symptom free at time of donation, was carrying a virus or infection that was not obvious.

Other risks that may derive from the FMT material itself may be unknown and expand as more is discovered about what gut bacteria influences. For example, in one case, an obese donor may have had the effect of weight gain on a recipient who gained weight following treatment. There are also case studies of a person becoming leaner after getting a transplant from a lean donor. But other factors may have affected these outcomes. However, since this is unknown territory, you may want your donor to be as physically and mentally fit as possible in addition to having been tested for disease.

THE FIRST PUBLIC STOOL BANK

OpenBiome was founded in 2012 by Mark Smith, a microbiology student at MIT, and James Burgess, an MBA student at the MIT Sloan School of Management. A family member of the two friends was seriously ill and suffered through eighteen months of agony from a C. diff infection. After he was unsuccessfully treated with seven rounds of Vancomycin, (a strong antibiotic), he finally received a life-saving fecal microbiota transplant.

In an effort to give more people access to this treatment, after much research and assistance from the MIT labs, they opened the first public stool bank in the USA. It has resolved many of the obstacles in providing physicians with quantities of reliably tested, healthy stool. Since its inception, OpenBiome has shipped over 20,000 transplants for use by medical providers. They are working with 800 providers in forty states in the US.

A quote from Smith and Burgess explains: "Motivated by the frustration of watching our friend struggle to access this effective treatment, and by scientific curiosity about FMT's potential, we founded OpenBiome in late 2012. We wanted to help make FMT safe and accessible for patients with recurrent C. difficile infection, and to give more clinicians access to the carefully screened samples necessary to perform FMT."

Despite the apparent safety of FMT and the obvious need for it, there was no easy way for physicians and clinicians to obtain enough screened donors and transplants for C. diff, patients and for clinical trials. Open Biome filled that need and today is the largest public stool bank in the US.

At the time of this writing, OpenBiome was supporting 14 enrolling clinical trials and in the planning and development stage of more than 35 other trials across a broad array of indications. Open Biome only sells to medical practices and researchers. The cost per transplant is approximately $200 each. Unfortunately, they cannot sell to individuals.

The same frustration and sense of urgency that inspired these two students to start OpenBiome still exists in the public domain. Despite its 98% rate of cure for C. diff. and its safety record, especially when compared with the negative health effects of multiple doses of strong antibiotics, it is still difficult for patients to find out about fecal transplants, to share this information with their doctors, who often have no experience with FMT, and convince them to perform this therapy.

Immunocompromised Patients

What about people who have been seriously ill and are in a weakened state? Colleen Kelly, M.D., a gastroenterologist in the Center for Women's Gastrointestinal Medicine at the Women's Medicine Collaborative, located in Providence, Rhode Island, conducted a multicenter study designed to answer this question. She identified eighty patients (including five pediatric patients) from sixteen different centers. All were immunocompromised patients from multiple bouts of C. diff.

Following FMT treatments, full resolution of C.diff infections and release from the hospital, none had infections or adverse effects related to the FMT treatment. "Researchers have found that fecal transplantation is effective and safe even for treating C. difficile in immunocompromised patients." The study, entitled Fecal Microbiota Transplant for Treatment of Clostridium Difficile Infection in Immunocompromised Patients, has been published in the *American Journal of Gastroenterology*.[16]

In one of the largest, if not the largest FMT study conducted, the Open Biome Stool Bank of Sommerville, Massachusetts in the US, studied results of 2,050 C.diff patients in multiple medical settings. The reported clinical cure rate from physician reported data using all delivery methods and all patient populations was 84.0%. In this study, no adverse effects (AE) were determined to be definitely related to FMT, 3 were possibly related and 39 not related to FMT based on

NIH criteria. Their conclusion based on these results were that: in "a large, real-world patient cohort that includes severe and refractory CDI patients, FMT from a public stool bank can be a safe and effective treatment for CDI not responsive to standard therapy."[17]

CHAPTER FOUR

The Gut and the Brain

Gut Feelings, Gut Instinct

Why do we *feel* things in our gut? Why do we often *go with* our gut instinct? When we are emotionally hurt, why do we feel like we were *punched in the gut?*

Since language was first written, human beings have described feelings emanating from our "gut." That sense of something being not right, an instinct pushing us in a direction we might not logically go, and that feeling was identified as coming from a place just below the stomach. Where do these feelings come from? Are they to be listened to? There was never any logical reason for these sensations to be coming from the intestines, right? I mean, the head, the heart, maybe, but the gut? We did not know then what we know now.

Bacteria and the Brain

Up until recently, it was thought that the gut and the brain were such separate systems that they could not possibly have much influence on each other. Then it was found that communication exists between the brain and the gut using neural, hormonal and immunological pathways. Called the enteric nervous system (ENS), it is comprised of two thin layers of more than 100 million nerve cells that line your gastrointestinal tract from the esophagus to the rectum. It interacts with the central nervous system (CNS) by regulating brain chemistry and influencing neuro-endocrine systems associated with stress response, anxiety and memory function. And that brings us back to "poop."

"You wouldn't believe what we're extracting out of poop. We found that the guys (bacteria) here in the gut make neurochemicals. We didn't know that." This is Mark Lyte, a researcher at Texas Tech University Health Sciences Center in Abilene, Texas in 2006 talking about his work.[18]

The neurochemicals, dopamine, serotonin and gamma-aminobutyric acid (GABA) are best known for their role in regulating emotions: arousal, inhibition, excitement, depression, happiness and anger. They are the neurotransmitters that create the pathway of communication from the gut to the brain. The gut also produces enkephalins (a member of the endorphins family) and benzodiazepines, the family of psychoactive chemicals that produce drugs like Valium and Xanax.

We had always assumed that these chemicals- the basic building blocks of our social behavior, mood, appetite and digestion, sleep, memory and sexual desire and feeling, were all in our heads. Or at least, all manufactured in the brain. In addition to all the higher functions, like thinking, they also are messengers that tell your heart, lungs and stomach to do their thing. Without them, life stops. They are critical components to mental and physical functions.

The gut has been called "the second brain" by gastroneurologists (those who study the interaction of the brain and the gut,) like Michael Gerson, Chairman of the Department of Anatomy and Cell Biology at New York–Presbyterian Hospital/Columbia University Medical

Center. Gershon, author of the book, *the Second Brain* (Harper Collins 1998) is considered a top expert in this new field.

Gershon clarifies this by adding that the second brain (also known as the enteric nervous system) does not help with conscious, complex thought processes but may be more a part of emotional thinking. "A big part of our emotions are probably influenced by the nerves in our gut," says Gershon. Emotional well-being may rely on messages from the "brain below" (in the gut) to the brain above. Our emotions are basically, a bunch of chemicals, ebbing and flowing like a tide in our bodies. Good mental health could be considered a state in which all the chemicals are in the right amount and type, all in balance. Without these neurochemicals, there are no emotions.

We like to think that our emotional experiences are coming from our big head brain, from rational thought, but evidence shows that the chemicals that create emotion are coming from the "second brain," the gut. Not only that, but about 90 percent of the communication flows not from the big brain down to the gut brain but vice versa. It is the gut sending out the majority of messages up to the head. The brain in the head is following commands from the gut, not the other way around. *Even more humbling is the knowledge that the lowest forms of life on earth, the bacteria in our gut, produce those very chemicals that control our emotional states.* The implications of all this on contemporary psychology are immense.

Neurotransmitter Depletion and Mental Health

For years, medicine has known that low levels of serotonin and/or norepinephrine can cause many diseases and illnesses. Now, it's known that aproximately ninety percent of the human body's total serotonin comes from the cells of the GI tract, where it is used to regulate intestinal movements. It is also active in the central nervous system where it regulates mood, appetite, and sleep. Serotonin impacts on some cognitive functions, including memory and learning. Many major antidepressants work by regulating levels of serotonin. Some of the diseases and/or illnesses caused by or associated with levels of serotonin and/or norepinephrine include: depression, anxiety, panic attacks, insomnia, migraines and other neurological conditions.

Serotonin seeping from the second brain might even play some part in autism, the developmental disorder often first noticed in early childhood. Gershon has discovered that the same genes involved in synapse formation between neurons in the brain are involved in the digestive tract synapse formation. "If these genes are affected in autism," he says, "it could explain why so many kids with autism have GI motor abnormalities" in addition to elevated levels of gut-produced serotonin in their blood.[19]

Bruce Lydiard in discussing the prevalence of psychiatric disorders among patients with irritable bowel syndrome in his article for the journal *Behavior Research and Therapy*, says: "Since the largest source of neurotransmitters is the gastrointestinal tract, it seems only right that digestive dysfunction and neurological conditions would go together. It is not surprising that intestinal disorders are found in high correlation with mental health conditions. These can include congestive bowel toxicity, Candida/yeast overgrowth conditions, increased intestinal permeability (leaky gut syndrome) and inflammatory bowel disease."[20]

Dopamine

Dopamine is another significant neurotransmitter produced in the gut and is implicated in many major mental disorders. Too high or too low levels of dopamine can be devastating to the functioning of the mind. Bi-polar disorder, psychosis, paranoia and schizophrenia all have higher dopamine levels than control subjects. Many of the major antipsychotic drugs reduce dopamine levels. However, too low levels of dopamine are also a problem as low levels are associated with depression, ADHD, addictions, and Parkinson's disease.

Since serotonin and dopamine are so intimately involved in mental health, is it possible that depression is merely too few neurotransmitters? Is schizophrenia merely too many? In animal studies, the addition of certain strains of bacteria brought about reversal of symptoms for autism, depression, anxiety and schizophrenia-like symptoms. *And if that were the case, then can addition of various strains of bacteria stabilize neurochemical production in humans and thus prevent or reverse mental illness?*

Multiple studies addressing these questions appear to answer this question positively. For example, Stephen Collins, a gastroenterology researcher at McMaster University in Hamilton, Ontario, has shown in his experiments that strains of two bacteria, lactobacillus and Bifidobacterium, can bring about a reduction in anxiety-linked behaviors in mice.[21]

Elaine Hsiao and other researchers reported in the journal *Cell* in 2015 that bacteria-free mice produced approximately 60 percent less serotonin than did their peers with conventional bacterial colonies. When these germ-free mice were recolonized with normal gut microbes, the serotonin levels went back up—showing that the deficit in serotonin can be reversed. "EC cells (enterochromaffin cells) are rich sources of serotonin in the gut. What we saw in this experiment is that they appear to *depend* on microbes to make serotonin," said Hsiao.[22]

Depression and Probiotics

Probiotics are used to introduce bacteria strains into the body and there is a lot of research studying whether improving our gut bacteria via probiotics affects our emotions and mental health. Chronic fatigue syndrome, (a disorder in which depression is a common symptom,) seems to improve with fecal transplant. It also apparently responds to probiotics. In a study of thirty-nine patients diagnosed with chronic fatigue syndrome, participants received either 24 billion colony forming units of Lactobacillus casei strain Shirota (LcS) or a placebo daily for two months. Patients provided stool samples and completed the Beck Depression and Beck Anxiety Inventories before and after the intervention.

Researchers found a significant rise in both Lactobacillus and Bifidobacteria in those taking the Lactobacillus casei, and there was also a significant decrease in depression and anxiety symptoms among those taking the probiotic vs controls.[23]

In 2016, a meta-analysis of multiple randomized, controlled trials of the use of probiotics for clinical depression was completed. The study reviewed 96 published papers and narrowed that down to five clinical trials involving 183 cases and 182 controls. The authors reported: "We found that probiotics were associated with a significant reduction in depression, underscoring the need for additional research on this potential preventive strategy for depression."[24]

The discovery of the size and complexity of the human microbiome has resulted in a complete reevaluation of the importance and impact of the gut-brain connection. Emeran Mayer, in his summary of scholarly works on the topic of gut microbes and the brain, published in 2014, said: "A growing body of preclinical literature has demonstrated bidirectional signaling between the brain and the gut microbiome. While psychological and physical stressors can affect the composition and metabolic activity of the gut microbiota, experimental changes to the gut microbiome can affect emotional behavior and related brain systems. These findings have resulted in speculation that alterations in the gut microbiome may play a pathophysiological role in human brain diseases, including autism spectrum disorder, anxiety, depression, and chronic pain."

What's in our gut apparently has a lot to do with how neurologically healthy we are. While we think our feelings, desires, reactions and decisions are under the control of our rational brain, we may actually be at the mercy of chemicals produced by "good" and "bad" bacteria within us.

In the next chapter, we will look at the role of bacteria in a modern epidemic, autism.

HOW BACTERIA AFFECTS BRAIN DEVELOPMENT

Recent studies with mice would indicate that not only does the microbiome produce the chemicals needed for the brain to function- but that the very development of different parts of the brain are dependent upon gut bacteria to grow to its full potential. Four parts of the brain were studied in bacteria-free mice. Each of the four parts showed a lack of normal development with consequential behavioral abnormalities. (But, it should *not* be implied from this that the brain cannot change or continue development later when the microbiome changes or other factors intervene.)

Striatum: In mice without bacteria, the flow of neural messenger's dopamine and serotonin is altered in the striatum, a brain area involved in movement and emotional responses. New connections may form more readily in the striatum too. These changes may cause bacteria-free animals to move and explore abnormally.

Hippocampus: Involved in memory and navigation, the hippocampi of germ-free mice have reduced levels of molecules that sense serotonin and the growth-related protein: brain-derived neurotrophic factor. These mice display memory problems.

Amygdala: Germ-free mice have changes in the levels of serotonin, BDNF and other signaling molecules in the amygdala, a brain structure involved in emotions. These alterations might contribute to an increase in risk-taking behavior.

Hypothalamus: In germ-free mice, the brain's stress responder, the hypothalamus, shows boosts in corticotropin-releasing factor and adrenocorticotropic hormone in germ-free mice. The changes might be related to the animals' heightened stress responses.

ref: S.M. Colllns M. Surette And P. Berciknat. rev MicroBlol. 2012

CHAPTER FIVE

Autism and Gut Bacteria

The Increase in Neurological Disease

Noting the prevalence of Alzheimer's disease, most of us are aware that brain diseases have increased in recent years. But, a British report published in 2015 showed that deaths due to brain disease in the United States have not just increased but exploded in numbers. Since 2013, death from a variety of brain diseases increased a huge sixty-six percent in men and an incredible ninety-two percent in women. The lead author in this study, Colin Pritchard, stated: "We need to recognize there is an epidemic that clearly is influenced by environmental and societal changes."[25]

In addition, one in six adults in the US suffers from a diagnosable mental disorder. These are shocking statistics and ones that should demand a focus on causes not just treating symptoms.[26]

As heartbreaking as Alzheimer's is when it appears in the elderly, it is even more horrendous to see young children, who seemed to be developing normally, suddenly lose the ability to communicate and relate to their loved ones and retreat into the shell of disability called autism that can destroy what was once a promising life.

Increase in Autism

In 1995, less than one child out of 500 in the US developed symptoms of autism spectrum disorder (ASD) as they grew. In 2000, that rose to about five in 1,000. Then the rate continued to rise alarmingly each year until it reached its current rate of one in sixty-eight children developing autism.

In looking for answers, scientists turned to genetics. But genetic changes take generations to occur. The rate of increase of this disorder was too fast and so it fits the category of epidemic. Interestingly, the rate of autism varies widely among countries. For example, in South Korea it is a frightening one in thirty-eight babies born. Some have pointed out that if these rates were to continue, autism could wind up being the *norm*, not the exception.

Another interesting feature is that autism rates among families who have immigrated from African, the Caribbean and other third world countries, to more developed western countries like Canada, the United States and Great Britain are much higher than rates in both their home country and higher than rates among citizens of their adopted country. Some immigrant families have multiple children on the ASD spectrum. In the Public Broadcasting System (PBS) documentary, *the Autism Enigma*, we meet several families of Somalian origin who migrated to Canada and gave birth in their new country to multiple children with autism. In Stockholm, Sweden, the prevalence of autism associated with learning disability was found to be three to four times higher among Somali children compared with other ethnicities in the city.[27]

This was affirmed by a study published in the *Journal of Pediatrics* June 2014, by the Fielding School of Public Health at UCLA. Studying the birth records of 1.6 million children born in Los Angeles County between 1995 and 2005, they identified 7,540 who were diagnosed with autistic disorder between ages three and five, and found information on their mothers' race, ethnicity and place of birth on their birth certificates.[28] Risk of autistic disorder was seventy-six percent higher in children of black foreign-born mothers, compared with children of white, U.S.-born mothers. It was forty-three percent higher in children of mothers from Vietnam, twenty-six percent higher in children of mothers from Central or South America and twenty-five percent higher in children of mothers from the Philippines. The risk was about thirty percent lower among children whose mothers were born in China or Japan.

This information reinforces the hypothesis that environmental elements (like dietary changes, for example) rather than genetics are the cause of ASD.

Autism and the Gastrointestinal System

While researchers began to look for environmental causes, physicians began to notice that these children had significantly larger problems with digestion, food allergies and sensitivities, diarrhea, enzyme dysfunction, leaky gut, and abdominal pain than the general public. That, plus all the information coming out of universities and research facilities revealing new roles of our gut bacteria, led to the idea that autism and other neurological diseases may be influenced or even caused by gut bacteria imbalances.

Multiple studies, including that of Dr. James B Adams of Arizona State University in 2011, in a study of fifty-eight children with autism spectrum disorder, found that gastrointestinal symptoms were strongly correlated with the *severity* of autism. In other words, the more severe the stomach issues, the more serious were the symptoms of autism.[29]

In the same year, in a study of 385 children, similar results were found. Author Andrew Wakefield said, "In a systematic analysis of an unselected population of 385 children on the autistic spectrum, clinically significant gastrointestinal symptoms occurred in forty-six percent compared with ten percent of the ninety-seven developmentally normal pediatric controls."[30]

In 2016, a meta-analysis of journal articles regarding this topic was published in the *Journal of Pediatrics* by Barbara McElhanon, MD & William G. Sharp, PhD. Their study found fifteen substantial articles on the topic. Their conclusion was "Results indicate greater prevalence of GI symptoms among children with ASD compared with control children." In fact, children with autism are about four times more likely to experience gastrointestinal (GI) distress than are their typically developing peers. The new analysis looked at data from 15 studies, totaling 2,215 children with autism and 50,664 controls. It found that children with autism are more than three times as likely to have diarrhea or constipation and more than twice as likely to feel abdominal pain than controls.[31]

So, there is a relationship between the health of our gut bacteria and disorders like autism. If that is the case, is autism ever reversible? Apparently, in some cases it is.

IS AUTISM REVERSIBLE?
THE ELLEN BOLTE STORY

Another key event that led researchers in the direction of a gut-brain connection in autism was the experience of Ellen Bolte. A Chicago computer programmer and mother of three,

Ellen Bolte was "delighted" with her fourth child, Andy. He was perfect, normal in every way, until, at eighteen months, he developed an ear infection. His pediatrician prescribed antibiotics. As the infection kept coming back, repeated courses of antibiotics were given.

Then Ellen began to see changes in Andy. Her previously cuddly baby refused to make eye contact, stopped vocalizing, and began to scream at everything. She says that his bowel movements were of a substance she had never seen before, he vomited mucus. His personality changed completely and everything seemed to be falling apart for him. He was losing his skills, "As my husband and I would put him to bed, we would ask ourselves, 'What did he do today that he won't be able to do tomorrow?'" Bolte said.

This occurred in the mid-nineties, before autism became a household word. At age two, Andy was given the diagnosis of autism. Andy's doctor insisted that Andy must have been born with the disorder and that it was genetic. But Ellen felt from watching Andy that he had *developed* autism following the ear infections. She began her own research. She took videos of Andy and kept very detailed notes and searched for a pediatrician who knew more about autism than she did.

Ellen sought help from over forty physicians including numerous specialists. None could give her any answers. Finally, Richard Sandler, a gastroenterologist, listened. He agreed to put Andy on a trial of Vancomycin. For one month, Dr. Sandler and Ellen documented changes in Andy. They videotaped his behavior at different stages and took notes. The first month was so productive and promising, Dr. Sandler agreed to a second month. But after that they knew they had to discontinue the antibiotic as long-term use can have serious negative effects. They wanted to advance their exploration and they contacted

Dr. Sydney Finegold of UCLA Medical center who was already working on the role of gut bacteria and how it affects behavior. He suspected that the bacteria that was at fault was Clostridia difficile, bacteria normally found in our bodies that, when allowed to run amuck, can cause serious infections and death.

He listened to Ellen's story and built a clinical trial based on the premise that Clostridia difficile (C.diff) bacteria are at fault in ASD. To test his theory, he worked with ten children who were autistic including Andy. He had "blinded" psychologists observe and take notes on behavioral changes and videotape the children every day. He administered oral Vancomycin, a strong antibiotic, the one typically used in treating Clostridia bacteria.

When antibiotics are given to treat a problem, like Andy's ear infection, they kill off a great deal of the good bacteria as well as the bad. Especially in cases where that bacteria (like Clostridia) is already resistant to antibiotics, the "bad" bacteria flourishes and takes over the entire digestive tract. Dr. Finegold's thought was that in Andy's case, the antibiotics for his ear infection had allowed the strong, drug resistant Clostridia to proliferate. Clostridia bacteria are known to produce metabolites that can directly affect the brain and behaviors. Vancomycin is one of the few drugs known to be effective against Clostridia.

Actual footage from Ellen's videos of Andy at different stages of development and then during and after his trial with Vancomycin can be seen in *the Autism Enigma*. In the videos we see Andy as a normal, playful baby, beginning to speak. Then, at about age two, after the course of antibiotics for his stubborn ear infection, he is seen to be clearly and severely autistic. Then you see him on film while on the Vancomycin. He is a different child, calm, vocalizing, trying to make contact with others, able to sit still and look at books, with no screaming.

And it wasn't just Andy who changed. Eight of the ten children "recovered" from many of their autistic symptoms including being able to sit still, vocalize and make eye contact with others. It was amazing and gave hope to all involved.

In the video, you can see the obvious joy in Ellen Bolte's face as she plays with her son. But you cannot keep a child (or adult) on that antibiotic forever and the spores of Clostridia are immune to antibiotics, so, following the end of treatment, it returns and with it, tragically, all the behaviors of autism. The last videos taken during the trial, weeks after the Vancomycin was stopped, show the Andy's return to the closed world of autism.

Specific Differences in Gut Bacteria in Children with Autism

The study that Dr. Finegold conducted, was aimed at children with regressive autism. That is, the child developed normally to a certain age and then "regressed" or lost previously gained developmental skills.

In testing the gut bacteria of these children, Dr. Finegold found that the fecal flora of children with regressive autism, compared with that of control children, had much higher Clostridia counts. The number of Clostridia species found in the stools of children with autism was greater than in the stools of control children. Children with autism had nine species of Clostridium not found in controls, whereas controls yielded only three species not found in children with autism.

Reasons to consider that microorganisms may be involved in late-onset autism include the following: (1) onset of the disease often follows antimicrobial therapy, (2) gastrointestinal symptoms are common at onset and often persist, (3) other antimicrobials (e.g., oral vancomycin) may lead to a clear-cut response and relapse may occur when the vancomycin is discontinued, and (4) some patients have responded to several courses of vancomycin and relapsed each time it was discontinued.

Per Dr. Finegold, "the issue can be raised as to whether the effectiveness of vancomycin might be related to some unknown property of the drug aside from its antimicrobial activity (e.g., an effect on the CNS). Because vancomycin is only minimally absorbed when given orally, it is much more likely that the effect is mediated through its activity on intestinal bacteria."[32]

The findings of this study, published in the *Journal of Child Neurology* in 2000, were major in the history of autism. They connected autism with the Clostridia bacteria and showed that the disease was not necessarily a permanent condition.[33]

Based on later clinical trials, published in the *Journal of Clinical Infectious Disease* in September 2002, Dr. Finegold formulated a probiotic treatment for certain neurological disorders including autism. He applied for a patent in 2004 based on that treatment.[34,35]

This important study was not given a great deal of attention because at that time it was believed that the gut and brain did not communicate. But discoveries that there was indeed a gut brain pathway and communication in recent years reopened this line of investigation. We now know that chemicals produced in the gut can make their way into the brain and that in actuality most of the neurotransmitters the brain uses are in fact produced in the gut.

OTHER AUTISM RECOVERY STORIES - THE JOHN RODAKIS STORY

Ellen Bolte's son is not the only case of temporary recovery from autism. There are others. One well-known case is that of John Rodakis, founder and CEO of N of One, an autism research foundation. Rodakis had two children, one of whom was diagnosed with autism. This child had been developing normally until about the age of two. His change in behavior was sudden and startling to his puzzled parents. He lost all desire to be held. He had difficulty making eye contact, rarely spoke and now refused to socialize with other children. They had a diagnosis that gave no hope for change or recovery.

In 2012, his two children came down with strep infections. Their pediatrician prescribed amoxicillin, a common antibiotic. Within two days of starting the amoxicillin, Rodakis and his wife began to notice changes in their son. He could look them in the eye and express affection and amazed them when he began to speak in sentences for the first time in his life. They were making contact with him and were excited. John Rodakis began documenting what was happening on an autism app (Autism Tracker) that allows you to record behavioral changes. The changes were wonderful. "Each day, he seemed to get better; I had no idea what was going on," Rodakis said.[36]

But, as happened with Ellen Bolte's son, once the ten-day course of antibiotics was finished, the old symptoms returned. They lost most, but not all, of what they had gained. Rodakis could not find physicians to help him find out what this meant. So, with a background in molecular biology and a career in medical venture capital and technology investing, John Rodakis began the N of 1 foundation. An N of 1 trial is a clinical trial in which a single patient is the entire trial, a single case study.

The idea was that each person's experience was important, valuable information that could lend clues to the autism puzzle.

Rodakis continued his research, talking with other parents, searching through medical literature. He found that many other parents had experienced this spontaneous recovery during antibiotic use. Many parents also reported that their child had a temporary recovery from autistic symptoms while running a fever. As with the antibiotics, the improvement was lost after the fever abated. *The fact that antibiotic use and fever were curative, points to a live organism such as bacteria, virus or fungus being the causal agent.* Rodakis also noted that the signs of autism improved every time he took amoxicillin, but not while taking co-trimoxazole, a combination of two other antibiotics (amoxicillin and co-trimoxazole differ somewhat in the types of bacteria they target. So, the antibiotics used are very specific and the bacteria that these antibiotics trigger are also very specific.

"Many in the research community are now beginning to view autism as something more akin to a metabolic syndrome, one that the microbiome may play a role in," Rodakis said.

Bolte and Rodakis are two of the more famous cases of autism reversal- but there are other physician and parental anecdotal reports of temporary recovery during both high fevers and specific antibiotic use.

Diet and Autism

Diet is one possible way to affect gut bacteria populations. Parents dealing with autistic children already knew that many of their children had food intolerances. Building on this, casein free (milk protein), gluten free and soy free diets were developed. Some eliminated food additives, like food dyes and preservatives like propionic acid from the diet. The results were mixed, but then that would be expected as individual food intolerances vary.

When the diet is full of carbs and sugar, the gut bacteria gets out of balance. Fungal and yeast infections prosper, dominating and overwhelming the good bacteria. The results of this survey may support theories that the gut bacteria affect (and possibly are the cause) of brain diseases like autism.

In 2001, a review of the existing literature on the effect of diet in autism, researchers Reichelt and Knivsberg of Norway concluded that in the past twelve years, many studies of this dietary intervention (gluten and casein-free) have been published in addition to anecdotal, parental reports. "The scientific studies include both groups of participants as well as single cases, and beneficial results are reported in all, but one study. While some studies are based on urinary peptide abnormalities, others are not. The reported results are, however, more or less identical; reduction of autistic behavior, increased social and communicative skills, and reappearance of autistic traits after the diet has been broken," said Reichelt.[37]

In a 2009 article published in the Annals of Clinical Psychiatry, the same two authors, Reichelt and Knivsberg reported that "IgA antibodies against the proteins casein, gliadin and gluten are statistically increased in children with autism. And we show highly significant decreases after introducing a gluten- and casein-free diet with duration of more than one year." They refer to other studies where children who participated were followed for four years with continued improvement. We refer to previously published studies showing improvement in children on this diet who were followed for four years.[38]

*There is indication from these and other studies that **short-term diets, twelve weeks or less, show few changes in behavior but that diets maintained for more than a year showed significant changes** and that improvement was seen even four years later.*

The possible reversal of neurological symptoms with the administration of a specific bacteria was reported in the Journal *Cell* in June of 2016. In the study, "Microbial Reconstitution Reverses Maternal Diet-Induced Social and Synaptic Deficits in Offspring" authors, Buffington, et al., put pregnant mice on a specific diet which caused changes in the gut microbiome of their offspring. The result was mice who exhibited specific autistic symptoms. The mice refused the company of other mice and acted out other behaviors similar to autistic behaviors in humans.

When the mice were treated with the bacteria L. reuteri, bacteria that fights Streptococcus mutans and h. Pylori, their levels of oxytocin increased and normal social behaviors appeared. The conclusion of the trial was: "We propose that a carefully selected combination of probiotics may be useful as a potential non-invasive treatment for patients suffering from neurodevelopmental disorders including autism spectrum disorders."[39]

Another bacteria implicated in neurodevelopmental disorders is Bacteria fragilis. Studies conducted at California Institute of Technology by famous researchers, Paul Patterson, Elaine Hsaio and Sarkis Mazmanian, published in the journal *Cell* in 2012 and in 2013 showed that mice who had been bred and treated to show symptoms of autism had reversal of symptomatic behavior after administration of B. fragilis. Their conclusion was: "Taken together, these findings support a gut-microbiome-brain connection in a mouse model of ASD and identify a potential probiotic therapy for GI and particular behavioral symptoms in human neurodevelopmental disorders.[40]

The above studies, as well as parental reports and physicians case studies show a correlation between different kinds of bacteria and autism symptoms. Long-term dietary changes are one way to affect the amount and types of bacteria in the microbiome as well as probiotics, the administration of specific strains of bacteria and the use of fecal microbiota transplants.

Probiotics and Autism

In 2014, Mayer, et al, pointed out in his paper, Altered Brain-Gut Axis in Autism: Comorbidity or Causative Mechanisms, that because metabolic products of the gut microbiome have long been implicated as a possible cause of ASD symptoms, probiotic treatment may be of benefit.[41]

In 2013, Sarkis Mazmanian and Elaine Hsaio published a paper that showed that Bacteria fragilis reversed autism-like symptoms in tests performed with mice. A serum metabolite (from Clostridia difficile, the same bacteria that causes deadly infections) induces autism like behavior in mice. Treatment with Bacteroides fragilis stopped abnormal communicative and anxiety-like behaviors in the mice.[42]

Fecal Transplant and Autism

We are just beginning to identify the many strains of bacteria our bodies need to function, and that information is critical. However, it may be generations before we truly understand the complexity of interactions between bacteria in the gut and are able to match a specific bacterial remedy to specific disease states. A more effective way to ensure the right healthy mix is to take a sample from a healthy, well balanced and high functioning microbiome and implant it in the person who needs it.

Dr. David Perlmutter, is a well-known neurologist and author of several books on the relationship of diet, brain function, and the prevention of neurodegenerative disorders. In his book, *Brain Maker*, Perlmutter tells the story of his twelve-year old patient, "Jason" who had been diagnosed with autism. Jason also had a long history of multiple antibiotic treatments.

Dr. Perlmutter ordered a stool analysis which showed almost no Lactobacillus bacteria in his colon. He prescribed Vitamin D and oral probiotics. Jason improved. He had diminished anxiety, could finally tie his own shoes, and for the first time in his life, was able to spend the night away from home. His mother arranged for a course of fecal transplants for him at the Taymount Clinic in the United Kingdom. Jason was so improved, following his treatment, that his mother took videos of him and sent them to Dr. Perlmutter. The videos showed Jason speaking animatedly to his mother and then laughing as he jumped up and down on a trampoline, things he could never do before. He is a changed child, according to his mother. "He is now social, conversational and sings hymns in church."[43]

WHICH BACTERIA DO WHAT?

Pulling findings from the above studies and others, we see that researchers are matching specific bacteria (or the lack of it) to specific conditions like anxiety, OCD, autism and memory problems. Animal studies so far show that:

- Bifidobacterium, and Lactobacillus showed beneficial effects on anxiety and depression, Wallace, JK C, Milev R, **The effects of probiotics on depressive symptoms in humans: a systematic review**, *Annals General Psychiatry*, 2017; 16: 14.
- Bifidobacterium infantis, improved stress related immune changes and depressive behavior in studies. Evrensel A, Ceylan ME, **The Gut-Brain Axis: The Missing Link in Depression**, *Clinical Psychopharmacological Neuroscience*, 2015 Dec; 13(3): 239–24.
- Lactobacillius helveticus ROO52 reduced anxiety like behavior and memory dysfunction.

- Ohland, CL, et al., **Effects of Lactobacillus helveticus on murine behavior are dependent on diet and genotype and correlate with alterations in the gut microbiome,** *Psychoneuroendocrinology,* 013 Sep;38(9):1738-47.
- Lactobacillus rhamnous JB-1 and L.helviticus reversed stress-induced memory failure in mice. Cowan, CSM, Callaghan, BL, and Richardson R, **Lactobacillus rhamnosus** and **L. helveticus, The effects of a probiotic formulation on developmental trajectories of emotional learning in stressed infant rats,** *Translational Psychiatry,* 2016 May; 6(5): e823.
- A combination of eight probiotics patented as VSL # 3, reversed age-related memory deficits. Disrutti E, O'Reilly JA, Fiorucci S, **Modulation of intestinal microbiota by the probiotic VSL # 3 resets brain gene expression and ameliorates the age-related deficit in LTP,** *PLoS One,* doi: 10.1371/journal.pone.0106503. eCollection 2014.
- Bacterius fragilis reversed autism and schizophrenia type induced behaviors in animal studies. Gilbert, JA, Krajmalnik-Brown, R., Knight, Rob. et al., **Toward Effective Probiotics for Autism and Other Neurodevelopmental Disorders,** *Cell,* Volume 155, Issue 7, p1446–1448, 19 December 2013.

Two Studies of Fecal Transplant and Autism

Studies are being conducted at present to see if probiotics and FMT can make a difference in persons with autism. Two recently completed studies include the following:

Researchers at Ohio State University conducted a study of 18 children, ages 7-17, with moderate to severe autism and gastrointestinal problems. All were given a course of antibiotics, followed by bowel cleanse. Then they received both oral FMT capsules and enema FMT for two days. This was followed by oral administration of standardized human gut microbiota (SHGM) over a period of seven to eight weeks. Patients and families reported 82% improvement in gastrointestinal issues.

ASD-related symptoms also improved. The Parent Global Impressions-III (PGI-III) assessment, which evaluates 17 ASD-related symptoms, showed significant improvement during treatment and no reversion 8 weeks after treatment ended, the researchers report. Of note, there was a significant negative correlation between change in GSRS and PGI-III scores, which "suggests that GI symptoms worsen directly with ASD behaviors, and that these can be altered via fecal transplant."

"We were hoping for some improvement in GI symptoms but were surprised to see 80% improvement," Ann Gregory, one of the study's lead authors and a microbiology graduate student at the Ohio State University in Columbus, told *Medscape Medical News*. "Further, we were hoping for some improvement in autism symptoms and were pleased to see about a 25% improvement in only 10 weeks that remained after treatment stopped," she added.[44]

In a second small study of nine children with ASD, (and one twenty-one-year-old adult,) at the University of Calgary and Alberta Health Services, patients were given a course of Vancomycin, seven days later followed by both oral fecal capsules and enema transmission of FMT. This was repeated a second day. "While ASD symptoms were not changed in the twenty-one-year-old, they were markedly improved in younger subjects on a more long-lasting basis." Culture results on one child indicated large quantities of Clostridium bolteae associated with ASD symptoms, which was absent post FMT treatment.[45]

A Review of 150 Papers

In 2017, scientists from the US and China collaborated on a review of 150 papers on the topic of whether diet, probiotics and fecal transplant can bring about positive change in persons with autism spectrum disorder. Their comprehensive study concluded that alteration of the gut microbiome can reduce symptoms of ASD. "ASD is likely to be a result of both genetic and environmental factors" explains Dr. Li, one of the paper's authors. He explains that the environmental factors include the overuse of antibiotics in babies, maternal obesity and diabetes during pregnancy, how a baby is delivered and how long it is breastfed. All of these can affect the balance of bacteria in an infant's gut, and so are risk factors for ASD. "Efforts to restore the gut microbiota to that of a healthy person has been shown to be really effective," continues Dr Li. "Our review looked at taking probiotics, prebiotics, changing the diet—for example, to gluten- and casein-free diets, and fecal matter transplants. All had a positive impact on symptoms."[46]

It appears that while antibiotics may both precede and possibly cause the initial onset of autism via disruption of the microbiome, they can in some cases, eliminate autistic symptoms temporarily. While courses of antibiotics temporarily kill bad bacteria and allow the patient to regain function, when antibiotic therapy is discontinued, spores of the bacteria hatch out and autistic symptoms return. Multiple studies indicate that FMT, diet and probiotics can reduce autism symptoms in many patients, in some cases dramatically.

CHAPTER SIX

Digestive Disease and the Gut

Digestive Disease - What it's like to have inflammatory bowel disease

I meet Allie at her house. I am driving her to the doctor's office to have emergency surgery yet again for the anal fistulas that keep cropping up as a result of her ulcerative colitis. Anal fistulae originate from the anal glands which drain into the anal canal. If the outlet of these glands becomes blocked, an abscess can form. The body tries to create canals that extend to the skin surface to drain the pus. If it cannot, the abscess becomes larger and harder. They are excruciatingly painful and sometimes cause fevers.

The patient is sedated and the surgeon cuts open the abscess allowing drainage. He also puts in a seton, a silk or rubber thread that helps keep the opening to the exterior from sealing up. Allie now has five of these setons. She has been operated on seven times or more. She never knows when she may need another surgery.

We have to drive her van because it has a portable toilet in the back. We may have to stop on the way as her colitis causes unpredictable diarrhea.

She suddenly says in a panicked voice, "pull over, pull over, I have to go." I look for a place to pull over, hopefully somewhat secluded. We pull over and park. I wait while she uses the portable toilet. She cries the whole time as it is so painful.This can happen more than once on the way to the doctor's and on the way home as well. This has been her life for the last two years.

What's Going on Inside You

We rarely think about what's going on inside our stomach and intestines unless we get a stomach ache, cramps or other overt problem. Most of us would be pretty shocked to see a real-time picture of what's going on down there with all that tubing from the mouth to anus. It is sort of a living slinky that can tense up and shorten or stretch out and relax. Like the pythons you see on TV, it can expand and contract to accommodate what we are putting into it.

But when things go wrong, it can wreak havoc with your personal and public life. Conditions like ulcerative colitis, Crohn's disease, celiac disease, irritable bowel syndrome, gluten intolerance and various other food sensitivities can bring on bouts of painful cramping, flatulence, fatigue, bleeding from the rectum, constipation or diarrhea, (sometimes uncontrolled, with humiliating accidents in public.) They can ruin your career, make it impossible to work outside the home, wreck your dating life or your participation in sports. Imagine, if you will, not being able to take long car rides without a portable toilet in the back seat of your vehicle. Unbelievably, this is the situation for thousands of Americans.

Even if there are symptoms so minor that you ignore them, they can be doing damage to your stomach, esophagus, intestines, and colon, creating a platform for more serious disease that may require surgery such as an ileostomy or colostomy, sometimes resulting in you having a bag attached to your side for life. Or you may require nutritional feeding (due to malnutrition) via a "PICC line" (peripherally inserted central catheter) or feeding tube. Fistulas (deep seated infections that create tunnels to the exterior of the body and drain pus) will sometimes arise in conjunction with bowel disease. They can take years to cure.

Digestive disease can lead to malnutrition, osteoporosis (with resultant bone thinning), anemia and heart problems (if iron levels go too low) and other illnesses. Digestive issues, while often hard to diagnose, cannot be ignored without paying a price later.

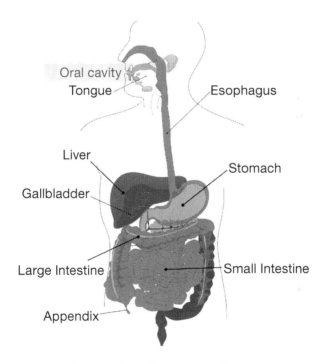

Copyright free photo per pexels.com

The Increase in Inflammatory Bowel Disease

In October of 2016, the CDC released a report stating that more than 3 million U.S. adults may have inflammatory bowel disease, according to a new government estimate. That's nearly triple the number of some previous estimates, the researchers said.

The new estimate is based on a national survey conducted by researchers in 2016, at the Centers for Disease Control and Prevention (CDC). Survey respondents were asked whether a doctor or other health professional had ever told them that they had either Crohn's disease or ulcerative colitis, which are the two types of inflammatory bowel disease (IBD). Based on the responses, the researchers estimated that 1.3 percent of U.S. adults, or 3.1 million Americans, have IBD.

"According to this report, the prevalence of IBD is much higher than previously estimated," says Dr. Siddharth Singh, a gastroenterologist and clinical assistant professor of medicine at the University of California, San Diego School of Medicine.[47]

An older report shows that this increase in bowel disease was happening with child populations even earlier, during the period 2002-2009. A report issued in the August 2013 print issue of the Journal of Investigative Medicine showed a *sixty-five percent increase in hospital discharges of children with the diagnosis of irritable bowel syndrome between 2000 and 2009*. The number increased from 11,928 discharges in 2000 to 19,568 discharges in 2009.

A comprehensive report on this increase and possible causes is summarized in this report in the *Saudi Journal of Gastroenterology*. "Over the last two decades, there has been a remarkable globalization of inflammatory bowel disease (IBD) with a striking increase especially in Crohn's disease. The relationship between genetics, microbiota, and environment are being unraveled at an exponential rate. The rapid increase of Crohn's disease point to significant globalized environmental contributions. The rising prevalence and incidence of IBD has been recently confirmed in a global systematic review."[48]

Differences in the Digestive Diseases

Defining and diagnosing these illnesses is difficult as there is considerable overlap in symptoms. Sometimes there are no overt symptoms until substantial damage has been done to the colon, intestines or stomach.

Irritable bowel syndrome (IBS) is a disorder characterized by abdominal pain or discomfort, and altered bowel habit (chronic or recurrent diarrhea, constipation, or both—either mixed or in alternation). Irritable bowel syndrome is a less serious but more common range of digestive problems. It is a group of symptoms but without any evidence of underlying damage.

IRRITABLE BOWEL SYNDROME STATISTICS

- IBS affects between 25 million and 45 million people in the United States. About two in three IBS sufferers are female. About one in three IBS sufferers are male. IBS affects people of all ages, even children.
- Worldwide it's estimated that 10-15% of the population has IBS.
- Most persons with IBS are under the age of 50. But many older adults suffer as well.
- IBS is unpredictable. Symptoms vary and are sometimes contradictory. Diarrhea can alternate with constipation. Long-term symptoms can disrupt personal and professional activities, and limit individual potential.
- Nearly 2,000 patients with IBS reported in a survey by International Foundation for Functional Gastrointestinal Disorders, (IFFGD) that diagnosis of their IBS was typically made *6.6 years after the symptoms began.*
- Approximately 20-40% of all visits to gastroenterologists are due to IBS symptoms.

These symptoms can occur over a long time, often years. IBS is classified into four main types depending on whether diarrhea is common (IBS-D), constipation is common (IBS-C), both are common (IBS-M), or neither occurs very often, but other symptoms are present (IBS). IBS negatively affects quality of life and IBS is a major women's health issue. Data reveals an increased risk of abdominal surgery in IBS patients. For example, 47-55% of women patients with IBS have had abdominal surgery of some kind, frequently ovarian surgery or hysterectomy. The cost to society, of IBS patients, in terms of direct medical expenses and indirect expenses from loss of productivity and work absenteeism is considerable, with estimates about 21 billion annually.[49]

Inflammatory bowel disease (IBD), on the other hand, is comprised of a more destructive group of conditions of the colon and small intestine. They are classified as autoimmune diseases, with Crohn's disease and ulcerative colitis being the two primary types. It is difficult for doctors to diagnose between the two without invasive tests but one main difference is that not only does Crohn's disease affect the small intestine and large intestine, it can also affect the mouth, esophagus, stomach and the anus whereas ulcerative colitis primarily affects the colon and the rectum. As opposed to IBS, people with IBD will show inflammation and damage to the colon and unlike IBS, IBD can be life threatening, usually from infections that occur from IBD.

Testing for Bowel Disease

Determination of specific bowel disease is made from tests such as endoscopy or colonoscopy. In endoscopy, a tube with a small camera is inserted down the throat while the patient is under sedation and the physician can examine- and sometimes treat-the esophagus, stomach, and upper part of the small intestine.

Endoscopes can also be passed into the large intestine (colon) through the rectum to examine this area of the intestine. This procedure is called sigmoidoscopy or colonoscopy depending on how far up the colon is examined.

As stated above, **Crohn's Disease** (CD) may affect any part of the digestive tract from mouth to anus. Symptoms include: abdominal pain, diarrhea, (which can be bloody,) fever and weight loss. Other complications can occur outside the gastrointestinal tract and include anemia, skin rashes, arthritis, inflammation of the eyes, and fatigue. Bowel obstruction can occur and Crohn's increases the risk of bowel cancer.

Approximately 780,000 Americans have Crohn's disease. It is most prevalent among adolescents and young adults between the ages of 15-35. In the years between 1992 and 2004, there was a seventy-four percent increase in doctor's office visits due to Crohn's disease. In 2004, Crohn's disease was the cause of 57,000 hospitalizations.[50]

Ulcerative colitis (UC), affects about 900,000 people in the United States. It is a long-term condition that results in inflammation and ulcers of the colon and rectum. The primary symptoms are abdominal pain and diarrhea mixed with blood. Symptoms come on slowly and can range from mild to severe. UC affects about 900,000 people in the United States. In any single year, about twenty percent of these people have moderate disease activity and 1 to 2 percent have severe disease activity, according to the Crohn's and Colitis Foundation of America.

Problems with Current Meds for Crohn's and UC and Other Digestive diseases

Currently, medications used for IBD fall into these categories: first: aminiosalicylates and corticosteroids which work by decreasing inflammation, second: immunomodulators that decrease the body's immune response and the newest class of drugs, biologics, which target specific proteins involved in the inflammatory response.

Some of these medications work by suppressing the immune system to stop it from over-reacting and attacking its own organs. This, while helpful, does not address the cause of IBD, nor does it cure it. It may put you into remission temporarily and that can be life-saving. But some of these medications also bring increased risk of infections and other aggressive diseases. Therapies that could address the cause of the disease and restore proper functioning of the immune system, however, would be more beneficial to the patient.

Fecal microbiota transfer, on the other hand, poses little risk, and aims to restore the health of the colon as well as the immune system. There is worldwide interest in the use of fecal microbiota transfer as therapy for disorders such Crohn's, colitis, celiac, and gluten and food intolerances. There are numerous clinical studies, clinical trials and case reports of FMT putting UC, Crohn's and other digestive disorders into temporary or permanent remission.

Can FMT be used as a treatment for Ulcerative Colitis and Crohn's?

In 2014, researchers R. J. Colman and D.T. Rubin of the University of Chicago's Inflammatory Bowel Disease Center found that while publications describing FMT as therapy for IBD more than doubled since 2012, research that studied FMT treatment efficacy was scarce. They decided to conduct a literature review and meta-analysis to evaluate the efficacy of FMT as treatment for patients with IBD. They included those studies in which FMT was the primary therapeutic agent and where clinical remission and/or mucosal healing were the outcomes. Here is what they found:

Eighteen studies were included. One hundred and twenty-two patients were described (79 ulcerative colitis; 39 Crohn's disease,

4 irritable bowel unclassified). Overall, 45% (54/119) of patients achieved clinical remission during follow-up. Among the cohort studies, the pooled proportion of patients that achieved clinical response was 36.2%

Their conclusion was that "FMT is a safe, variably efficacious treatment for IBD." They suggested that frequency of FMT administration, donor selection and standardization of microbiome analysis were factors that can affect outcomes.[51]

A more recent meta-analysis in 2016 of current literature and clinical studies of FMT for treatment of ulcerative colitis, included twenty-five studies with 234 ulcerative colitis patients. Overall, forty-one percent, (or eighty-four out of two hundred and two patients achieved clinical remission (CR) and sixty-five percent (or one hundred and twenty-six out of one hundred and ninety-three patients achieved clinical response. Adverse events were minimal and self-resolved. The analyses of gut microbiota in seven studies showed that FMT could increase microbiota diversity and richness, similarity, and certain change of bacterial composition.

The study authors concluded that "FMT provides a promising effect for UC with few adverse events. Successful FMT may be associated with an increase in microbiota diversity and richness, similarity, and certain change of bacterial composition."[52]

Longer Treatment Necessary for Ulcerative Colitis/Crohn's Disease

For infections like C.diff, one application of FMT seems all that is necessary for most patients. But clinical trials for UC and Crohn's show better results with more frequent administration over an extended time frame. As is shown in the example below, *six to eight weeks with administration five times each week has shown the best results for people with severe cases of ulcerative colitis.*

The study, presented at the European Crohn's and Colitis Organization 2016 Congress, showed that fecal transplants conducted over eight weeks on people with severe and resistant ulcerative colitis were "cured" of diarrhea and rectal bleeding. One of the principals on the study, Sudarshan Paramsothy, MD, from the University of New South Wales in Kensington, Australia, says it's the largest and most intensive trial of fecal transplants to treat colitis. All patients in the study had active mild-to-moderate ulcerative colitis and phased out the use of steroid treatment during the study period. In the study, 41 adults received a fecal transplant by colonoscopy, then followed up with five active fecal transplant enemas each week for 8 weeks, done at home. The test used 150 milliliters of fecal material from previously frozen stool from three to seven unrelated donors.

Another 40 received a placebo treatment. Of the forty-one patients receiving fecal transplants, forty-four percent were considered to be in remission without symptoms. That means they had no rectal bleeding or diarrhea. Only twenty percent of the placebo group achieved remission.

During a study extension, thirty-seven people in the placebo group chose to switch and receive fecal transplants.[53]

In these three studies referenced above, it is interesting to note that there was a consistent percentage of forty to forty-one percent clinical remissions and about sixty-five to sixty-six percent clinical responses in the two meta-analysis described above (Colman and Shi), which is close to the forty-four percent clinical remission found in the University of New South Wales, Australia study.

Methods of delivery, variety, quality and choice of donors, age and condition of recipients and most importantly, the number of transplants each participant received are all factors that can create variance in these results. Again, studies seem to show that higher success rates in treatment of colitis can be achieved with longer trials of say, eight weeks or more, in which the recipients are getting about five transplants a week. The success of the transplants is also dependent upon the amount of damage previously done to the colon by disease.

Gluten and Wheat Reactions

Wheat allergy is an allergic reaction to foods containing wheat, one of the top eight food allergens in the United States. A wheat allergy generates an allergy-causing antibody to proteins found in wheat. Typical symptoms are swelling, itching or irritation of the mouth or throat, hives, itchy rash or swelling of the skin, nasal congestion, headache, itchy and watery eyes, difficulty breathing, cramps, nausea or vomiting, diarrhea. Reaction can be severe as with anaphylactic shock.

Celiac disease (CD), is an autoimmune disorder (affecting primarily the small intestine) that occurs in people who are genetically predisposed. It is caused by a reaction to gluten, the proteins found in wheat and in other grains such as barley, and rye. With celiac, gluten triggers the immune system to attack the lining of your small intestine. The resulting intestinal damage, called villous atrophy, can cause malnutrition and conditions such as osteoporosis, iron deficiency and cancer.

Classic symptoms include gastrointestinal problems such as chronic diarrhea, abdominal distention, malabsorption, loss of appetite, and among children, failure to grow normally. There may be mild or absent gastrointestinal symptoms, a wide number of symptoms involving any part of the body, or no obvious symptoms. There is a blood test for celiac but the patient must be consuming gluten on a regular basis for the test to show antibodies.

Gluten intolerance or Non-Celiac Gluten Sensitivity

Gluten intolerance can display all of the same symptoms of celiac but will not show up in a blood test. It can be as destructive to the body as celiac and should be treated as seriously.

Celiac Disease is Increasing in the Population

Gluten intolerance is increasing in the population. One measurable way to see that is through blood tests given to new recruits for the army and air force. As it happens, both services test for celiac disease in their recruits and so extensive records are available that show the rate of increase in the population over the years.

In their 2009 study, doctors analyzed stored blood samples, taken from Air Force recruits in the early 1950s, for gluten antibodies. They assumed that one percent would be positive, which is today's rate. But they found instead, that the number of positive results was far smaller in the past, indicating that CD was a rarity at that time. They then compared those results with two more recently collected sets from Olmsted County, Minnesota. Their findings suggest that *CD affects roughly four times more people than in the 1950s.* Additional studies done later showed a five-fold increase from 1999 to 2008. "This tells us that whatever has happened with CD has happened since 1950," Dr. Murray, the lead researcher said. "It suggests something has happened in a pervasive fashion from the environmental perspective."

Dr. Murray was also concerned because as he says, "Only 1 in every 5 people with celiac disease will be diagnosed — the remaining four will elude diagnosis, so we're not doing a very good job of detecting it."[54]

Hiding in Plain Sight

Dr. Murray says the real problem in diagnosing celiac disease is that it is often hiding in plain sight. Although it damages the small intestine, CD can affect any part of the body, including the nervous, reproductive, endocrine, skeletal and cardiopulmonary systems. A substantial number of patients may not present with classic gastrointestinal symptoms, such as diarrhea, weight loss, bloating and abdominal pain, but rather with anemia, osteoporosis, peripheral neuropathy, ataxia or cognitive impairment.

With celiac, as opposed to other autoimmune conditions, the cause of the disease is well known; it is the ingestion of gluten. Why should a substance that we have been eating for centuries suddenly become a problem? And why should that problem be multiplying rapidly among Americans? People can argue that some digestive diseases were simply not diagnosed in the past, or that since the tests for them are so invasive that people refused to have them done. But celiac has been diagnosable with blood tests the army has been using for several generations so the pattern of increase is undeniable.

There is speculation that the increases may be explained by the progressive westernization of diet, the development in recent years of new types of wheat with a higher amount of cytotoxic gluten peptides, and the higher content of gluten in bread and bakery products, due to the reduction of dough. There is also speculation that the widespread use of genetically modified grains and the substantial amounts of pesticides and herbicides applied to grains may be causing reactions.

FMT and Celiac Disease

Some case histories and personal stories have shown that FMT can be helpful for overall food intolerance and general gut health, but, even so, celiac is a lifelong disease and once you have it, you will always have to stay on a gluten-free diet. Here is one man's testimony. Roger Elliot, a longtime celiac sufferer, who received two weeks of FMT treatment at the Taymount Clinic in England.

> *"Eight weeks ago, I went to the Taymount Clinic near London for their FMT treatment. I had been suffering from increasing food intolerances for over 10 years, and things had got to such a stage where I could only eat a highly-restricted diet.... In addition to this, I'm celiac, so all my food has to*

be scrupulously gluten free. The only thing that really made any difference to my health at any stage was moving to a paleo diet, but even then, I still continued to lose more and more foods. By the time I went to the Taymount Clinic I was pretty desperate because things had worsened to the point where I was starting to worry that I would soon have no foods I could eat without becoming ill. …..After the treatment, nothing seemed very different, I was still getting reactions to food …….But for the last six weeks I've been eating more and more foods, some of which I haven't eaten without being made ill for over 5 years. These are early days, ….. but I can't describe how it feels to have been given some respite from the situation I was in."

In this case, while FMT did not "cure" Elliot of celiac, it appears that it made him less sensitive to other foods.[55]

Tests for Celiac and Gluten Related Disorders

It is recommended that if celiac disease is suspected, that you do *not* take gluten out of your diet until you have had the blood test for it. If gluten has been out of your diet for a while, the test will be negative and then it might take 6-12 months of consuming gluten again to build up enough antibodies in your blood. Firm diagnosis is a positive blood test, followed by an endoscopy and biopsies. While you must stay away from gluten for the rest of your life, the damage done from gluten intake often can be remediated once the full diet is followed. This is not a diet you can cheat on because very small amounts of gluten can create big reactions. Gluten is found in any product with wheat, rye or barley flour including malt products, some alcohols, gravies, soups, toothpaste, skin creams and cosmetics. French fries in restaurants are frequently rolled in flour prior to packaging to keep them from sticking together. Ask before you order.

Unless a product is clearly marked gluten free, it may not be.

In addition to the blood test, a diagnosis can be reached by undergoing an endoscopic biopsy. This procedure is performed by a gastroenterologist as an outpatient procedure. A biopsy is taken of the small intestine, which is then analyzed to see if there is any damage consistent with celiac disease. The diagnosis may be confirmed when improvement is seen while on a gluten-free diet.

You can also try this: go off all sources of wheat and gluten. Check the ingredient labels on everything you eat for two weeks. Be especially careful eating out. Most restaurants have a gluten free menu. If it does not say gluten free assume it is not. After one week, note changes in how you feel and how your digestive system is working. Then eat a lot of wheat in one day and see if you react with stomach pain, diarrhea, constipation or other symptoms.

The only treatment for celiac disease or gluten intolerance is a lifelong, strict gluten-free diet. People living gluten-free must avoid foods with wheat, rye and barley, such as bread and beer. It is extremely important to avoid ingesting even small amounts of gluten as this may damage your intestines. Sources of gluten, can include products that are gluten free but manufactured in a setting that also processes wheat or gluten products and crumbs from a cutting board or toaster. FMT cannot cure celiac disease nor gluten intolerance but may make you less sensitive to other foods.

A condition that is implicated in food sensitivities is leaky gut.

Leaky Gut

Sounds gross, right? While you can't actually see this problem, researchers are thinking it may be a key link to how the digestive system initially starts to malfunction.

The only thing that separates your bloodstream from the messy contents of your intestines is a single layer of epithelial cells. This thin, flexible skin allows the absorption of nutrients while also functioning as a barrier, which stops antigens and pathogens from entering the blood stream. Joints and junctures at points along the membrane can be tightened or loosened depending on what body process is taking place. When the junctions fail to tighten, harmful substances (particles of food and other material) can leak into the bloodstream causing the body to react as though to an enemy invader, attacking its own tissues in an effort to rid itself of the foreign bodies. Leaky gut is also known as increased intestinal permeability or intestinal hyperpermeability.

Leaky gut is implicated in autoimmune, inflammatory, and allergic type diseases, which can manifest both locally (within the gut) and systemically throughout the body. So, dysfunction in the gut can then create problems in other parts of the body that are not even in contact with the gut, such as skin, lungs, joints.

Known conditions that co-exist with leaky gut are celiac disease, Crohn's disease, food allergies, type one diabetes and other autoimmune diseases, certain drug exposures, and radiation therapy. It is also suspected that exposure to glyphosate, the active ingredient in the herbicide *Roundup*, causes increased intestinal permeability.[56]

Glyphosate

This popular herbicide is so widely used in commercial farming that in the two states (Idaho and Mississippi) tested by the US Geological Survey Office, back in 2011, glyphosate was found in 75% of every water and air sample tested. In other words, people living in those areas were inhaling it as they breathed and drinking it in their water. Since 2011, use of glyphosate has only increased as it is now also used to hasten "ripening" of grain crops just before harvest.[57]

In an article published in 2013, in the journal *Interdisciplinary Toxicology*, it was noted that celiac disease is growing in numbers so that an estimated five percent of the population in North America and Europe now has this disease! The article proposes that glyphosate, the active ingredient in *Roundup* herbicide, is a primary cause of increases in gluten intolerance and celiac disease.

Glyphosate residue is found in almost all vegetables, fruits and grains available to us in our grocery stores unless organically produced and labeled as such. Glyphosate has been shown to inhibit the production of enzymes and vitamins and create deficiencies of needed minerals. In laboratory tests, glyphosate applied to intestinal tissue, can be seen to weaken and dissolve the tight junction intestinal barriers within sixteen minutes of application.[58]

It is probable that it is also in the air and water of other states where large scale farming is carried out. This herbicide could be responsible for decreased quantity and quality of gut bacteria in those who consume it, whether through oats, wheat, soybeans, edible beans, sugarcane, vegetables or other foods sprayed with *Roundup* or through exposure in the air or water. This could account for the increased numbers of people suffering from gut disease and the increasing numbers of cases of celiac disease and gluten sensitivity in this country.

Alessio Fasano, MD, a world-renowned pediatric gastroenterologist, research scientist, and founder of the University of Maryland Center for Celiac Research, believes **all autoimmune conditions have three factors in common: a genetic susceptibility, antigen exposure, and increased intestinal permeability.**

"Besides celiac disease, several other autoimmune diseases, including type 1 diabetes, multiple sclerosis, and rheumatoid arthritis, are characterized by increased intestinal permeability secondary to non-competent tight junctions that allow the passage of antigens from the intestinal flora, challenging the immune system to produce an immune response that can target any organ or tissue in genetically predisposed individuals," Fasano wrote in the February 2012 issue of Clinical Reviews in Allergy and Immunology.[59]

While it was previously believed that the autoimmune disease process remained ongoing once activated, if Fasano's statement is true, then the progress of autoimmune disease may be reversed by interrupting one of the three modifiable factors mentioned above. While genetic susceptibility cannot be altered, antigen exposure may be reduced by eliminating offending substances and intestinal permeability can be stabilized, this information should give hope to those with autoimmune disorders. Books such as *the Wahl's Protocol*,[60] by Dr. Terry Wahls, and Dr. Susan Blum's *The Immune System Recovery Plan*,[61] as well as the testimony of people who have had significant changes in their health due to major dietary changes or from FMT would indicate that this is the case.

What is Zonulin?

Zonulin (syn. Haptoglobin) is a protein that modulates the permeability of tight junctions between cells of the wall of the digestive tract.) Zonulin is normally present in the intestines to control the passage of fluids, macromolecules, and leukocytes, but this protein appears to be overexpressed in patients with autoimmune conditions, resulting in increased intestinal permeability. Fasano adds, "When the zonulin pathway is deregulated in genetically susceptible individuals, both intestinal and extra-intestinal autoimmune, inflammatory and neoplastic disorders can occur. It has been suggested that if the zonulin-dependent intestinal barrier function is restored, then these damaging autoimmune processes can be stopped."[62]

Gluten and Zonulin

According to this theory, improving intestinal permeability should be a focus for those with autoimmune disease. In people who are sensitive to it, gluten is one factor that can modulate zonulin secretion. Dr.

Fasano believes that, "Once gluten is removed from the diet, serum zonulin levels decrease, the intestine resumes its baseline barrier function, the autoantibody titers are normalized, the autoimmune process shuts off and, consequently, the intestinal damage heals completely."

In other words, increased intestinal permeability could contribute to the autoimmune response in predisposed individuals. Studies have shown that this process could be involved not only in celiac disease but also in a significant number of other autoimmune diseases. Abnormal intestinal permeability also has been shown to be present up to one year before a clinical flare-up of inflammatory bowel disease.

These are some startling considerations that directly connect gut health and activity with autoimmune disease throughout the body.

But what causes zonulin to increase and cause the subsequent leaky gut?

Dr. Zachary Bush, former Chief Resident for the Department of Internal Medicine at the University of Virginia and now in private practice in Charlottesville VA, says: "Environmental toxins, gluten, GMOs, commercial agricultural herbicides, and widespread antibiotic use in humans and in livestock damage the gut and allow these toxins to weaken the immune system. When these toxins leak out through the gut wall, the immune system breaks down, and the toxins can attack every organ in the body." So, elements in the environment weaken our guts, they malfunction and leaky gut begins. Then, as more and more trash leaks out of the intestines into surrounding tissue, the immune system begins to over-react targeting benign foods and attacking different body systems. Food sensitivities and allergies result. One or more of a host of autoimmune diseases begin to present themselves.

Solutions for Leaky Gut

Most health practitioners recommend taking these irritants out of your diet/life: refined sugars and carbohydrates (they encourage inflammation and growth of "bad" bacteria and yeasts, milk casein and gluten because so many people are sensitive to them, alcohol and NSAIDS (non-steroidal, anti-inflammatory drugs) because they irritate the stomach and gut lining. You should also check for infections like H.pylori and try to reduce your stress (mental, emotional, physical.)

Dr. Robynne K. Chutkan, MD, FASGE, Assistant Professor of Medicine, Georgetown University Hospital, Founder and Medical Director, Digestive Center for Women suggests that these steps may be helpful for leaky gut.

"An anti-inflammatory diet that eliminates refined sugars, dairy, gluten, alcohol and artificial sweeteners—some of the biggest offenders when it comes to inflammation—can be very helpful. Consuming lots of anti-inflammatory essential fatty acids in fish and nuts, and filling up on green leafy vegetables, high-fiber and fermented foods that help to promote the growth of good bacteria is also crucial." She adds that a strong, high quality probiotic can be an important addition and that glutamine has been shown in some studies to help with intestinal injury after chemotherapy and radiation and may be beneficial in leaky gut.

Doctor Chutkan warns it may take six weeks or more to see a change and it may take several months and even years to heal a damaged intestinal lining in extreme cases of leaky gut. Because we're still learning about leaky gut, many of the treatment guidelines are drawn more from anecdotal observation than from rigorous scientific studies. But they're sensible recommendations that can lead to improvements in your overall health, whether or not you have increased intestinal permeability.[63]

Summary

Italian researcher Francesca Mangiola said in a *World Journal of Gastroenterology* article in January 2016. "In the last few years, the importance of gut microbiota in the maintenance of the physiological state in the GI system is supported by several studies that have shown a qualitative and quantitative alteration of the intestinal flora in a number of diseases. The application of gut microbiota modulators, such as probiotics, antibiotics, up to FMT (fecal microbiota transfer), has been widely experimented as a therapeutic instrument for GI diseases with exciting results."[64]

This gives both patients and physicians a relatively safe, inexpensive and easily accessed direction to pursue in search of therapies for these conditions.

The Bigger Picture

Crohn's disease and colitis are classified as autoimmune diseases. Food intolerances and allergies may also be signs of immune system malfunction. In the next chapter, we will see how digestive disease fits into the larger picture of autoimmune disorders and why other autoimmune conditions may also have their origin in the gut.

CHAPTER SEVEN

The Rise of Autoimmune Disease

J ust as digestive diseases are epidemic, so are autoimmune diseases spreading at a rate not seen before. "One in twelve Americans— and one in nine women—will develop an autoimmune disorder."[65]

This shocking statement by Douglas Kerr, faculty neurologist and neuroscientist at the Johns Hopkin's Hospital in Baltimore, MD, is quoted from the foreword of the book *The Autoimmune Epidemic* by Donna Jackson Nakazawa.[66] It is reinforced by the National Institute of Health's estimate that, (as contrasted with the 13 million Americans with cancer,) up to 23.5 million Americans have an autoimmune disease and that those numbers are rising. In fact, autoimmune diseases are now among the top 10 leading causes of death in American women under the age of 65. (footnote)The American Autoimmune Related Diseases Association (AARDA) argues that true numbers of persons with autoimmune disease are much higher as autoimmune disease usually takes years to diagnose. They are estimating that the number of people in the US with diagnosed and undiagnosed autoimmune diseases is more likely to be fifty million.[67]

Internal Army, The Incredible Immune System

Our immune system is a fantastic network of communicating cells and organs, as constantly active as a hive of bees. Worker T cells, (white cells from the thymus gland,) distinguish between friend or foe microbes and B cells (bone marrow- or bursa-derived cells) and produce antibody fighters to attack the enemies. Together, they act as a defensive army launching attacks against invading pathogens. These enemies can include microbes and viruses that carry colds and flus, as well as more serious germs that can bring lethal diseases. Some cells of the immune system can even recognize cancer cells as invaders and kill them.

An especially important part of this activity is the T cell's ability to distinguish the difference between our own cells and foreign invaders. It is the failure of our T cells to make the distinction between our own cells and enemy invaders that is the foundation of most autoimmune disease. While the T cells come from the thymus gland, the gut plays an important role in training the T cells to recognize our own cells. In the gut, the white cells are changed from immature T cells into regulating T cells by friendly bacteria. The gut bacteria also produce immune-activating molecules called cytokines. Cytokines signal white blood cells to move towards sites of inflammation, infection and trauma. So, to have a "strong" immune system you need plenty of T cells and plenty of good gut bacteria to help them function.

Once it has been exposed to an invader, the immune system has the ability to remember that enemy and recognize it if it sees it again. This ability to quickly identify pathogens and remember how to attack them is why vaccines work. The principle behind vaccination is that if the body is exposed to a small dose of the offending substance, it then creates its own blueprint of attack, successfully defeats its foe and stores away that information. Then, when exposed to the same virus or germ again, it will recognize it and immediately take aggressive action using a predesigned plan of attack. This is also why populations never exposed to a pathogen before are much more vulnerable to it.

One reason that cancers are often hard for the immune system to fight is that cancers have a unique way of disguising themselves so that they look like a normal part of the body, a friend rather than an enemy. Many areas of cancer research are now working on finding ways to teach the body to tell the difference between a cancer cell and a normal cell.

But, sometimes the immune system goes haywire. It can become over-reactive to substances that are not naturally harmful. Things like pollen, animal dander, foods and medications for example. Those reactions become allergies. The body then remembers those items and continues to attack them every time they are present. Unfortunately, this pattern can also apply to the organs and tissues of our own bodies. Scientists believe that while genetics play a role, triggers such as environmental, chemical, stress, drugs and infection must also be present to initiate this destructive over-activity of the immune system.

The immune system may aggressively and relentlessly attack the joints to cause rheumatoid arthritis or destroy the myelin sheath surrounding the nervous system causing the devastating crippling of multiple sclerosis, or it can damage the beta cells in the pancreas which results in type I diabetes. These autoimmune disorders are numerous including: fibromyalgia, arthritis, chronic candidiasis, ulcerative colitis, Crohn's disease, food reactions, chemical sensitivities, rrheumatoid arthritis, systemic lupus erythematosus (lupus), inflammatory bowel disease (IBD), type I diabetes mellitus, Guillain-Barre syndrome, psoriasis and others. Autoimmune conditions are chronic and can affect every organ in the body, involving almost all medical specialties, including gastroenterology, cardiology, neurology, rheumatology, gynecology, dermatology, and endocrinology.

Where is the immune system located? We have learned that seventy percent or more of the immune system is located in the gut. "A huge proportion of your immune system is actually in your GI tract," says Dan Peterson, assistant professor of pathology at the Johns Hopkins

University School of Medicine. "For example, certain cells in the lining of the gut spend their lives excreting massive quantities of antibodies into the gut. That's what we're trying to understand—what are the types of antibodies being made, and how is the body trying to control the interaction between ourselves and bacteria on the outside?"[68]

The discovery that the gut is connected to the brain and has pathways to virtually all of the body made it plausible that the antigens produced in the gut could affect much more than just the digestive arena. The gut is, in fact, the central command for the entire immune system.[69]

This explosion of new knowledge shows that immune conditions share a common bond in the intestinal lining of individuals with autoimmune diseases, with these diseases often progressing for years before an obvious illness appears.

Since intestinal bacteria play such a critical role in maintaining proper immune system function, changes in that bacteria may be the cause of many inflammatory autoimmune diseases. Sarkis K. Mazmanian, professor at the California Institute of Technology" and international expert on gut bacteria has said: "It is conceivable that the absence of beneficial microorganisms (due to dysbiosis) that promote appropriate immune development leads to the inflammatory responses that underlie various immune diseases in humans."[70]

In numerous journal articles it has been suggested that if gut bacteria is the problem then probiotics, which feed and sustain microbial populations, may be of benefit for autoimmune and inflammatory diseases. And, any factor that can alter the gut microbiota balance, such as diet or antibiotic treatment, should be seen as a potential risk.[71]

Unfortunately, immune system disorders are studied and treated as separate specialties when the remedy for all may be a common one. That is, the proper feeding and maintenance of our intestinal bacteria.

Specific Autoimmune Diseases and FMT/Probiotics

In his article, Fecal microbiota transplantation broadening its application beyond intestinal disorders,which appeared in the *World
Journal of Gastroenterology* in January, 2015, author Meng-Que Xu,
listed those diseases (exclusive of digestive disease) associated with
gut dysbiosis and the research studies that made the connection.
It was a surprising list, including metabolic syndrome, cardiac
disease, Type II Diabetes, multiple sclerosis, Parkinson's Disease,
non-alcoholic fatty liver, autism, chronic fatigue syndrome, lym-
phoma, mammary tumors, arthritis and various allergic disorders
including asthma.[72]

Most of these are classified as autoimmune and many others on
the list are possibly in that category. Comprehensive in its coverage of
international studies related to FMT, it painted a picture of just how
far reaching the effects of our bacteria are and how important FMT
may be now and in the future.

Beyond those studies mentioned in Meng-Que Xu's article, there
are numerous case studies, reports and clinical trials involving a
wide array of immune related diseases and the use of either fecal
microbiota transfer or probiotics (or both) available online and at:
https://clinicaltrials.gov.

Here is a small sampling.

Multiple sclerosis (MS) is an autoimmune disease that begins
when the T cells cross into the central nervous system and set about
attacking the myelin coating around nerve fibers.

Symptoms usually come on gradually with minor problems with
stiffness, mobility, balance. There may be bowel or bladder dysfunction, speech or swallowing problems. But as time goes on, they become
severe enough to cause concern and then the diagnosis is made. MS
is a terrible disease that can eventually rob you of the ability to walk,
drive, control your bathroom functions and many other losses of
ability that are life destroying.

The Multiple Sclerosis Foundation estimates that more than 400,000 people in the United States and about 2.3 million people around the world have MS. About 200 new cases are diagnosed each week in the United States. Rates of MS are higher farther from the equator.[73]

Is gut bacteria different in MS patients?

A research team from Weill Cornell Medical College and the Rockefeller University has identified a bacterium it believes may trigger multiple sclerosis. A study of MS patients found that they had ten times the antibodies to epsilon toxin as did people without MS. It also showed that only 23% of the MS patients had A Bacterium in their stool. A Bacterium is protective in the body against colonization by Epsilon Toxins. The implication might be that without the proper bacteria (in this case A Bacterium) destructive bacteria (Epsilon Toxins) are able to rampantly multiply and produce metabolites that initiate diseases like MS.

The team also examined stool samples from both MS patients and healthy controls enrolled in the HITMS clinical study and found that 52 percent of healthy controls carried the A subtype compared to 23 percent of MS patients. "This is important because it is believed that the type A bacterium competes with the other subtypes for resources, so that makes it potentially protective against being colonized by epsilon toxin secreting subtypes and developing MS," say Rumah and Vartanian, who headed the study.

"One of my favorite approaches is development of a probiotic cocktail that delivers bacteria that compete with, and destroy, C. perfringens types B and D," Vartanian says. "It would be such a beautiful and natural way to treat the gastrointestinal system and solve the problem. We are also starting to work on this approach."[74]

"A growing body of evidence has implicated the human gut microbiome in a range of disorders, including obesity, inflammatory bowel diseases, and cardiovascular disease. Animal studies present compelling evidence that the gut microbiome plays a significant role in the progression of demyelinating disease, and that modulation of the microbiome can lead to either exacerbation or amelioration of symptoms. Differences in diet, vitamin D insufficiency, smoking, and alcohol use have all been implicated as risk factors in MS, and all have the ability to affect the composition of the gut microbiota. Preliminary clinical trials aimed at modulating the gut microbiota in MS patients are underway and may prove to be a promising and lower-risk treatment option in the future."[75]

FMT & MS

Three case studies of individuals with multiple sclerosis, who underwent FMT for constipation, achieved normal bowel function and also experienced a long-standing remission in MS symptoms, were reported in a paper by Thomas Borody, Medical Director of the Center for Digestive Disease in Sydney Australia.

His three cases are submitted here as he reported them:

> Case 1: A 30-year-old male with constipation, vertigo and impaired concentration and a concomitant history of MS and trigeminal neuralgia. Neurological symptoms included severe leg weakness and he required a wheelchair and an indwelling urinary catheter. Previous failed treatments included Mexiletine, Tryptanol and 9-interferon. The patient underwent 5 FMT infusions for his constipation, with its complete resolution. Interestingly his MS also progressively improved, regaining the ability to walk and facilitating the removal of his catheter. Initially seen as a 'remission', the patient remains well 15 years post-FMT without relapse.

Case 2: A twenty-nine-year-old wheelchair-bound male with 'atypical MS' diagnosis and severe, chronic constipation. He reported parasthesia and leg muscle weakness. The patient received 10 days of FMT infusions which resolved his constipation. He also noted progressive improvement in neurological symptoms, regaining the ability to walk following slow resolution of leg parasthesia. Three years after the patient maintains normal motor, urinary and GI function.

Case 3: An eighty-year-old female presented with severe chronic constipation, proctalgia fugax and severe muscular weakness resulting in difficulty walking, (diagnosed as 'atypical' MS.) She received five FMT infusions with rapid improvement of constipation and increased energy levels. At eight months she reported complete solution of bowel symptoms and neurological improvement, now walking long distances unassisted. Two years post-FMT, the patient was asymptomatic.

Conclusion: "We report reversal of major neurological symptoms in three patients after FMT for their underlying GI symptoms. As MS can follow a relapsing-remitting course, this unexpected discovery was not reported until considerable time had passed to confirm prolonged remission." These cases were reported initially on Dr. Borody's website and other cases involving remission of auto immune diseases have been published on this website since.[76]

Another case is that of a forty-three-year-old MS patient ("Carlos," not his real name) who sought help for chronic constipation at the Taymount Clinic in the UK. At the time he attended he could barely walk with the help of a cane. After receiving fecal transplant there, not only was his constipation resolved but his MS symptoms were, in his own words, "sixty percent cleared." He regained the ability to walk unattended. (Read his first-person report on the Taymount Clinic website: taymount.com.)

Rheumatoid Arthritis

Arthritis refers to inflammation in the joints. **Rheumatoid arthritis** is a severe form of arthritis that occurs when the immune system begins to attack the joints. It affects joints on both sides of the body, such as both hands, both wrists, or both knees and can result in malformed hands, wrists, etc. RA can also affect the skin, eyes, lungs, heart, blood, or nerves.

A thirty-one-year-old woman with rheumatoid arthritis transitioned her whole family to a gluten-free diet when her three- year-old daughter was diagnosed with celiac disease.

At the mother's follow-up visit with her rheumatologist, her doctor remarked on the significant reduction in her C-reactive protein and erythrocyte sedimentation rate levels, two inflammatory markers indicating disease activity in rheumatoid arthritis (RA.) The mother reports she wakes up pain-free every morning since starting a gluten-free diet.[77]

Researchers already are aware that the gut microbe mix of those with rheumatoid arthritis is different. "Patients who first develop rheumatoid arthritis have substantially lower number of helpful bacteria in their gastrointestinal systems.[8] People with rheumatoid arthritis have significantly less Bifidobacteria, Bacteroides-Porphyromonas-Prevotella species, Bacteroides fragilis species and the Eubacterium rectale-Clostridium coccoides species."[78]

"It's been suspected for years and years, that the development of autoimmune diseases like arthritis is dependent on the gut microbiota" Diane Mathis, professor of microbiology and immunology at Harvard Medical School, in Boston, Mass who was not involved in the work, told Science NOW. It's a very striking finding, she said.[79]

Parkinson's

In a recent *Cell* publication, a team led by Timothy Sampson and Sarkis Mazmanian of Caltech showed that gut microbiota can promote inflammation of neurons and motor deficits in a human α-synuclein mouse model of Parkinson's disease. The germ-free mice who received transplants with the human gut microbiota from patients with Parkinson's disease displayed a significant worsening of the hallmarks of Parkinson's disease, whereas those receiving fecal transplants from healthy human donors did not show the symptoms.[80]

Chronic fatigue syndrome (CFS) is a disorder characterized by extreme fatigue or tiredness that doesn't go away with rest and can't be explained by an underlying medical condition. The fatigue is so severe that it renders patients exhausted much of the time. There are other symptoms ranging from insomnia, easy bruising, swollen lymph nodes, vertigo, and sensitivity to cold, heat, light and sound. Depression is another major symptom.

Two studies show that differences in the intestinal flora have been observed in patients with chronic fatigue syndrome. In one study of thirty-nine individuals with CFS,[81] the proportion of gram-negative Escherichia coli was reduced in CFS patients versus that in healthy controls (49% versus 92.3%).

A study in 2013[82] examined a larger group of 60 CFS patients with gastrointestinal symptoms who had undergone FMT. The results showed that seventy percent of patients responded to treatment and fifty-eight percent retained complete resolution of symptoms during a fifteen to twenty-year follow-up period.

Allergic disorders

As with immune disorders, allergies have been increasing in modern society, particularly over the past 50 years. A current hypothesis suggests that the disruption of intestinal microbiota initiates allergies.

Multiple studies have been conducted with humans and mice to determine the relationship between allergic diseases and microbiota.

Mice raised germfree, that is with no exposure at birth to bacteria from a mother and none from subsequent exposures as they grow, develop more severe allergic disease than conventional mice. In addition, early-life antibiotic exposure seems to be related to the development of allergy related asthma and food allergies.[83]

It may be that many autoimmune diseases are created by an imbalance of gut bacteria with one or more species (or the lack of a certain species) being the cause.

CONNECTION BETWEEN INFLAMMATION AND THE IMMUNE SYSTEM

Paul O'Toole is a professor at the Alimentary Pharmabiotic Centre, which is part of the BioSciences Institute at Cork, Ireland. His research has been focused on finding ways to reduce problems of aging like muscle loss (sarcopenia), and cognitive decline. Many of these age-related problems are caused by chronic inflammation. O'Toole explains that significant links have been established between gut microbiota and inflammation, sarcopenia and cognitive function. "Inflammation," he says, "is not a swollen thumb. *Inflammation means how activated your immune system is.*" The gut bacteria, responsible for the healthy functioning of the immune system, can be the cause of excess inflammation in the body. As the body ages, the microbiome decreases in quantity and variety. So, increasing the variety of foods you eat and perhaps adding probiotics may be two ways to reduce inflammation and slow the aging process.

The Immune System, Cancer and Fecal Microbiota Transplant

Bacteria in the gut has been implicated with several forms of cancer, notably, colon cancer. But now, more studies are showing that good gut health can have multiple effects on prevention and treatment of many kinds of cancer.

As stated in her article, Gut Microbes, Diet and Cancers, Meredith Hullar Ph.D, of the Fred Hutchinson Cancer Prevention Center in Seattle Washington says: "An expanding body of evidence supports a role for gut microbes in the etiology of cancer. Previously, the focus was on identifying individual bacterial species that directly initiate or promote gastrointestinal malignancies; however, the capacity of gut microbes to influence systemic inflammation and other downstream pathways suggests that the gut microbial community may also affect risk of cancer in tissues outside of the gastrointestinal tract."[84]

In addition to initiating inflammation and producing toxins, an imbalance of bacteria can cause the immune system to malfunction, leaving us open to malignancies that otherwise would be destroyed by the activity of our T cells and B cells.

Cancer is a difficult disease to treat because it can appear to be normal cells, hiding its true identity from our defending T cells. When that happens, "checkpoints" stop our immune system from attacking the cancer. Checkpoint inhibitors are new form of chemotherapy that help your body recognize malignancies and open the "checkpoints" so our T cells can go on the offensive.

Scientists were puzzled by the fact that some patients responded remarkably well to treatment with checkpoint inhibitors and went into remission. But some patients did not. What was making the difference?

Jennifer Wargo of the MD Anderson Cancer Hospital in Texas, was studying this problem with melanoma patients. She had read studies by two separate researchers who had already demonstrated you could improve a mouse's response to checkpoint inhibitor therapy by giving him certain types of bacteria. So, she collected stool samples from 300 cancer patients who then received checkpoint inhibitors as treatment. The results were night and day. The patients who had a higher diversity of gut bacteria had a stronger response to checkpoint inhibitor therapy. Her conclusion was that: "Melanoma patients' response to a major form of immunotherapy is associated with the diversity and makeup of trillions of potential allies and enemies found in the digestive tract."[85,86]

Another study, found that patients who had recently been given antibiotics did not respond to chemotherapy as well as did patients who had not had antibiotics prior to chemo treatment. The study concluded that antibiotics destroy favorable gut bacteria and reduce the functioning of the immune system, thus reducing the efficacy of the immunotherapy.[87]

"Ultimately, doctors might be able to reduce a person's risk for cancer by analyzing the levels and types of intestinal bacteria in the body, and then prescribing probiotics to replace or bolster the amount of bacteria with anti-inflammatory properties," said Robert Schiestl, professor of pathology, environmental health sciences and radiation oncology at UCLA and the study's senior author.[88]

Putting it all together

With our new-found knowledge of the relationships between our microbiome, immune system and our brain we can ask the following question:

Is it possible that changes in our diet, grains, food crops, environmental assaults from antibiotics, chemicals such as herbicides, pesticides, plastics, air pollution, have deteriorated our gut bacteria and resulted in never before seen increases in neurological disease, digestive disease and autoimmune disease? Can it be that our guts are so defunct we can't protect ourselves anymore from various cancers, viruses and pathogens? Even worse, it may be that our malfunctioning immune systems have turned against us causing an onslaught of diseases like multiple sclerosis, Parkinson's, lupus, Crohn's Disease, ulcerative colitis and celiac.

CHAPTER EIGHT

The Causes of Gut Failure

THE AUTHOR'S STORY

My story begins when at age 15. My mother, in a desperate attempt to improve my teenage life, took me to a dermatologist to be treated for acne. Pimples were the bane of my existence, making me even more awkward and shy than I was to begin with. The doctor put me on antibiotics, tetracycline- I think, to start. It worked pretty well. He also gave me "lamp treatments" and told me to get as much sun as possible. No mention of sunscreen or skin cancer.

But as months went by, I began to get more and more severe acne and cysts. He upped the dosage of antibiotics, switching types and dosages to more potent types. Months became years and I found I could not get off of the antibiotics without having more serious infections. Every winter was a series of colds. Every period I had brought on massive candida infections. Still the antibiotics were increased. I knew something was wrong but had no idea what to do about it.

When pregnant with my first child, I went off of antibiotics and was sick throughout the pregnancy. I lost 30 pounds from my normal weight and looked like I had been in a concentration camp. I was terrified my child would be malnourished. When I finally gave birth to a normal weight, seemingly healthy baby, I was relieved. But when I nursed him, I was appalled to find out that I could not breast feed him as I infected him with thrush, (a fungal infection in the mouth) each time I nursed him. Years of antibiotics had given me a persistent candida (yeast) infection.

In his first year, my son seemed to do well, except that he was hyperactive. He could not take a nap and had great difficulty sleeping at night. Caring for him was extremely exhausting and more than one sitter I hired quit because his energy level was too much. He began to experience stomach aches and severe hyperactivity. Milk seemed to be a problem, but his pediatrician insisted there was no such thing as milk allergy. I realized he was reacting to foods and had a hyperactive reaction in particular to food dyes. One dose of red cherry soda could easily keep him awake for 24 hours. He lost weight and his white cell count was so low they believed he might have leukemia. I was terrified.

A turning point occurred when an elderly neighbor said to me: "Get that child some raw goat milk from the country- that will turn him around." And it did. I found a retired sheriff who raised long-eared goats. On a diet free of food dyes and cow's milk, and fortified with raw unpasteurized goat milk, he thrived, gained weight and his white cell came back to almost normal. I found out later that he had multiple food allergies and chemical sensitivities.

In the meantime, I continued to have fungal infections every month when I had my period. By pure chance, a book was published *around that time with the title: The Yeast Connection, by William G. Crook, MD. It explained everything. The antibiotics over the years had destroyed all my good bacteria which allowed the candida to flourish. The next ten years or so was followed by monthly doses of antifungal drugs such as Nystatin and then Nizoral, then Diflucan to combat the monthly yeast infections each time I had a period. When these yeast infections occurred, I often had patches of what looked like athlete foot fungus on various parts of my body as well as a roaring vaginal yeast infection and a general flu-like feeling. My immune system was marginal as was my son's. Every fall and winter were filled with constant bouts of strep throat, colds, and, in many years, pneumonia.*

As time progressed and I went through menopause, I was delighted to find that the monthly candida bouts also disappeared.

But then, I began to have occasional episodes of diarrhea. After a year or so, they increased in frequency, becoming a major nuisance in my life. I also found that my stomach became too sensitive to tolerate alcohol or acidic foods.

I had unrelenting diarrhea off and on for four years. Despite seeing two GI docs and having a colonoscopy, there was no diagnosis, just the medical bills. I mentioned it to my new gynecologist who said "try going off of gluten for a week and see what happens. Half of my patients are gluten intolerant." I did and was amazed. While I still had watery, loose stools, the unrelenting diarrhea was finally gone.

During those four years I had also been diagnosed with early onset osteoporosis and been put on at least three medicines which resolved nothing. I also had surgery for appendicitis and developed cysts on my liver, pancreas and ovary. Most worrisome of all, a blood test marker (CA 19-9) for pancreatic cancer came in at twice the normal level. My belief is that gluten intolerance and the resulting digestive failure caused malabsorption and inflammation.

After two years of eating gluten free, I had a bone density test performed. The technician came back and said, "We have to repeat the test, this can't be right. Bone density doesn't improve this much, especially at your age." I had grown new bone in the areas previously tested. She repeated the test and told me the osteoporosis was reversed and asked me what I had done. The gluten-free diet had allowed my body to rebuild lost bone.

While the diarrhea was mostly resolved, I continued to have occasional problems with it. During this time, a friend recommended a product that had helped her called "Restore." Specifically designed to tighten the junctures in the intestines and resolve leaky gut. Within twenty-four hours of taking a teaspoon of this product I had the first well-formed stool in over four years. So, a gluten-free diet and a leaky gut product solved a four year plus problem that was ruining my health.

The Garden of the Gut

Think of a garden. A garden with thousands of different varieties of miniature plants. Greens, greys, fluorescent yellows, pale greens, rich purples, shades of mahogany, burgundy, carmine reds, golden yellows, dark thick foliage, with an endless variance of geometric and asymmetric designs in its branches stems and flowers, all of it tiny, microscopic, no end to the eye's delight in the variety of form and color. So amazing. This sunless garden can be flourishing; feeding on abundant nutrients and moisture, constantly in motion, absorbing and then releasing powerful chemicals, like flowers producing pollen, that will travel all the way to the brain (and other organs) making the whole machinery of the body work in perfect harmony.

To thrive, this garden needs pure, clean water, free of contaminants. It needs a sleep period to restore itself. It needs a wide variety of foods with good quantities of minerals and vitamins. It needs unique nutrients to produce its wide variety of bacteria.

But then, if the garden is flooded with herbicides, sanitizers, and bacteria-killing chlorine (not to mention antibiotic medications—the nuclear "herbicide" of the gut garden), some species will die, never to return. If it is fed materials with little nutritional value, the garden may become sickly, losing its color and vitality, hanging on but functioning only minimally. The garden produces less nutrients and vitamins. Parts of your body begin to suffer. Impairment of the digestive system begins. The gut makes less neurotransmitters. The immune system starts to malfunction. The wonderful chemistry of the body breaks down. Disease results, and over time, finally the whole organism is at risk.

This is your gut bacteria. And, in a broad sense, it can be said that the same things that impact our whole body, in a good or bad way are also impacting our gut health. The air you breathe, the water you drink, the food you eat, the amount of sleep you get and even, according to one study, exercise, all affect what's happening in your gut.

The following are hypothesis on the cause of gut failure and represent the thoughts of prominent researchers internationally.

Antibiotics

The most common cause of gut failure is the use of antibiotics. Some types of antibiotics target only certain species of antibiotics. Others kill good and bad bacteria indiscriminately. While they can be life-saving, antibiotics should be used with caution. Their effects on the microbiome are drastic and difficult to remedy. Studies have shown that up to half of the bacteria in the gut can be destroyed from one course of antibiotics and can take months to recover, if ever. A good reason to go organic is that antibiotic residue is found in our poultry, beef, pork, eggs and milk.

Once Gut Bacteria is Lost, it's Hard to Get Back

We know that when we take antibiotics, we wipe out amounts of both good and bad bacteria in our microbiome. Will this regrow on its own? And if so, how long does it take? While answers to these questions are highly variable between individuals, two studies on this topic have shown that it can take a much longer time than was previously thought.

David Relman and Les Dethlefsen of Stanford University, using a technique developed by Mitchell Slogin of the Marine Biological Laboratory in Woods Hole, MA, were able to identify changes in the gut microbial communities of three healthy people after taking the antibiotic Ciproflaxin for five days. The scientists were able to identify roughly 3,300 to 5,700 different types of bacteria in the human gut and found that the antibiotic treatment affected about of a third of the identified bacteria. They also found that while some of the "good" bacteria came back—some didn't, even six months later. So, how to get rid of the bad bacteria and replace the lost good bacteria and make that change more stable?[89]

Air Quality

While genetics and diet have been looked to as primary causes of many digestive diseases, we are now realizing that the air we breathe has a far greater impact on this system than was ever imagined. Multiple recent studies are studying the effects of air pollution not only on the lungs and cardiovascular system but on gut bacteria as well.

"We tend to think about air pollution in terms of lung health, but the GI tract is also being bathed in it continuously. Fine pollution particles are cleared from the respiratory tract by mucous that makes its way to the gut," said Karen Madsen, a gastroenterological scientist from the University of Alberta in Edmonton, Canada. The route of contact is either as mucous cleans particles from the lungs or dietary intake of food and drinking water, contaminated with particulate matter from the air. Once in the intestines, the particles will have both direct effects on bowel disease (IBD), irritable bowel syndrome, and enteric infections in infants. The gut microbes also turn the particulate matter into toxic metabolites that act as poisons and create more damage to the intestinal system.[90]

The study concludes that the ingested matter can trigger and accelerate development of inflammatory digestive disease, especially in genetically vulnerable individuals.

Another study found a link between smog and appendicitis. Elevated levels of ozone, the main ingredient of smog, were linked to an increased risk of a burst appendix in a study of more than 35,000 people across twelve Canadian cities between 2004 and 2008. Researchers in these studies believe that gut bacteria is ultimately what is being affected by the pollution. "In the gut, you have a barrier between the immune system and the bacteria that live there. It's important that barrier gets maintained," Madsen, one of the leaders of the study, said.[91]

In a later study, Kaplan, part of the same team as Mardsen, said: "Understanding the risk factors can help us to mitigate the risk and prevent people from getting the disease in the first place." Some evidence suggests inhaling fine particles, or soot, may disrupt the immune system and trigger inflammation in the gut by making it more permeable and altering its normal bacteria.

Another study by Kaplan and colleagues found that people in the United Kingdom, between the ages of 5 and 23 with higher exposure to nitrogen dioxide, a component of traffic exhaust, were more than twice as likely to develop Crohn's disease as young people with less exposure.[92]

It is frustrating to think that not only do we have to pay for purified water because our natural sources are polluted, but that the very air we breathe is also contaminated, yet that is a sad fact that cannot be ignored.

Water

The American Water Works Association says that chlorination of water has, by itself, extended the lifespan of Americans by fifty percent in the last century. It has almost eliminated water-borne illnesses such as typhoid fever and cholera. But while chlorine is killing off those bad microbes it may be also killing off the good ones. While there are no studies to look at, it's an easy call to make. Chlorine was meant to kill microbes and it does that without prejudice. We really do not know all the ramifications of chlorine in our water supply.

Today's water supplies vary widely in quality. As we saw in Flint Michigan, you really don't know what is in your water supply unless you have it tested by a reputable lab. Chemicals that have leaked from fracking sites, mining operations, chemical plants and underground gasoline storage tanks all contribute to making our water supplies unhealthy. Not to mention the pesticides, herbicides, and household chemicals that are flushed into our water systems. The best answer is an inhouse filtration system. You can also get an attachment for your shower that filters out the chlorine.

Sleep

A very small study conducted in 2017 at Uppsala University in Sweden links lack of sleep, (even over as short a time as two days,) with the loss of almost fifty percent of the bacteria in the gut. Participants in the study were given eight and a half hours sleep for the first two days at a sleep facility. The next two nights they got only four and a half hours of sleep while a control group had the usual eight and a half hours. Specialized testing of stool samples showed a fifty percent drop in bacterial cultures in the sleep deprived group.

A secondary finding of this study was that the participants were also found to be twenty percent less receptive to insulin after two nights of sleep deprivation, and interestingly, their gut flora then mirrored the gut flora of previously observed subjects who were either clinically obese or had metabolic disorders. Lack of sleep has long been linked to obesity. However, it has never fully been understood exactly how the two are linked, other than that disturbed sleep seems to reduce our cells sensitivity to insulin. This puts a huge burden on the body as more and more insulin is needed to regulate blood glucose levels, which may eventually lead to the development of either type two diabetes or obesity.[93]

Exercise

We know that exercise is the answer to just about everything, so it should not be a surprise that it affects gut bacteria as well. A study, conducted with the National Rugby Team of Ireland and researchers at University College Cork, defined at least one kind of bacteria that thrives in a well exercised body.

The athletes in this study had a significant difference in their gut bacteria as compared to two sets of control groups. (One, a group of similar age men who exercised moderately and the second, consisted of same-age couch potatoes.) The rugby players had considerably more diversity in the make-up of their gut microbiomes, meaning that their intestinal tracts hosted a greater variety of germs than did those of the other men, especially the sedentary group.

Specifically, the rugby players' guts harbored larger numbers of akkermansiaceae, bacteria associated with a decreased risk of obesity and very low systemic inflammation. The men who rarely exercised had relatively small numbers of the same bacteria as well as elevated markers for inflammation in their bloodstreams. These findings "draw attention to the possibility that exercise may have a beneficial effect on the microbiota," Dr. Shanahan, leader of the study, said.[94]

Hygiene Hypothesis

A current theory, especially in the allergy and immunology field, is the "Hygiene Hypothesis." In previous times, children growing up had extensive exposure to the soil. Home gardens were in every backyard. Children played in the dirt, made mud pies (and sometimes ate them.)

Today, we sterilize and sanitize everything, including our children and food. As we became increasingly civilized, we began to buy all our foods and our milk from large producers. In previous decades, foods were grown, harvested and often fermented in homes and small farms. Yeasty breads, pickled vegetables, sauerkraut, cheeses, home-made wines and beers, all contributed to a wide diversity of microbes in our bodies. Fermented foods containing all kinds of "good" bacteria were common in most households. Milk was unpasteurized exposing children to even more bacteria. While breastfeeding has made a comeback, for some generations and for many contemporary moms, formulas take the place of breast milk.

The speculation is that the lack of exposure to infectious agents, microorganisms (such as the gut flora or probiotics), and parasites, increases susceptibility to allergic diseases by suppressing the natural development of the immune system. In other words, we are not exposed to a wide enough range of pathogens and end up with an overreactive immune system.

Western Pattern Diet

Also called the "Standard American Diet" and the "Sweets and Meat Diet," the Western Diet is one that is high in animal products, sugar, and flour and low in raw foods, especially vegetables. It lacks whole grains and fiber, has an overabundance of simple sugars and is loaded with things that are likely toxic to both the garden and its soil- the mucus. (Emulsifiers destroy the mucus layer in which the bacteria live.) This diet favors dysbiosis of the gut by providing opportunity for "bad" bacteria, yeast, and other pathogens to get the upper hand. Today's frequent carbo-centric meals continuously feed the bad guys who then overwhelm the good bacteria.

Environmental Factors

In addition to the types of foods we choose to eat, widespread use of hormones, herbicides and insecticides *on* the food all add to damage to the gut by killing, reducing or increasing various kinds of microbes. The previously mentioned condition, leaky gut, can result from these toxic exposures and cause deterioration of the digestive system. Genetic modifications of foods open another Pandora's Box of possibilities regarding gut imbalance and damage.

Gut Infections

Thankfully, our gut is naturally resistant to infection by pathogenic bacteria, due to acid produced in the stomach that is designed to kill potential invaders. But, due to the ease of global travel, we are now exposed to numerous new creatures from all over the globe. Germs, viruses and other bacteria our systems have never had contact with are interacting with our over-burdened and weakened guts and gut ecosystems. Aspects of our modern diet and lifestyle including chronic stress and use of acid-suppressing drugs have compromised our defenses. Several types of gut infections have been linked to IBS. For example, food poisoning caused by Blastocystis hominis, Dientamoeba fragilis, and giardia bacteria leads to chronic, persistent IBS in as many as ten percent of cases. Intestinal parasites like lamblia may be relatively common (yet often undiagnosed) causes of IBS, even in the developed world.

All of this information may be overwhelming in its application. Purified water, filtered air, organic fruits and vegetables, gluten-free foods may all seem like just too much effort. But here is the good news. Attention paid to all these things not only contribute to your general health and energy, they reduce your risk of today's common, scary, and costly illnesses, including cancer, autoimmune disease, and cardiovascular disease.

CHAPTER NINE

How to Make Gut Bacteria Thrive

Helping Gut Bacteria Thrive

The importance of temperature, oxygen levels, quality of the water and soil, the bad bugs, the good bugs, the pollinators, the fertilizer, all of these have parallels in the gut. While we have centuries of knowledge about gardening, we know relatively little about the gut garden. But every day, there is yet another discovery revealing something new about how the gut functions and the microscopic creatures who run it. You know some of the things that can kill the plants and creatures in your garden. Here are some things you can do to help it flourish. As mentioned in the previous chapter, clean air, clean water and enough sleep are all basics of building a good gut.

Get Dirty

Speaking of soil, Dr. Robin Chutkan's book, *The Microbiome Solution*, talks about getting dirty as a way of helping to build a robust microbiome. This is in sync with the "hygiene theory" of why we are having such an increase in autoimmune disease: Too many antibiotics in our foods and medicines, too many antimicrobial cleaners, mouthwashes and hand sanitizers, too many pesticides and herbicides found in our food and water.[95]

Some of Dr. Chutkan's recommendations include: don't use products that have chemicals such as: petroleum products, FD&C dyes, fragrances, parabens, phthalates, sodium laurel sulfate, triclosan, triethylamine, or other harmful chemicals. Don't use microbial cleaners, hand sanitizers, bleach, antiperspirants, or mouthwash as they can alter your microbiome. She points out that the skin is permeable and whatever goes on your skin goes into the body.

Where can you find products to use that are free of chemicals that are harmful? The boom of natural food stores is a response to that need. Most grocery chains now have aisles of natural or organic products. Farmers markets are a great place to find real probiotic foods with the right stuff. And online you can get just about anything you need.

She suggests that it's a good thing to get your hands dirty gardening, to play in the mud, to have plants and open your windows to put you and your family more in touch with a variety of microbes.

Variety in your Diet

Glenn Taylor, director of the Taymount Clinic in England, famous for his work with bacterial transplants, says one of the most important aspects of diet and bacteria is variety in the diet, "Variety on the plate equals variety in the gut.

He suggests keeping a list of every food, herb, spice, beverage and condiment you eat in a week. He says you should be able to see at least fifty different foods in that one week. It's not as hard as it seems. He also states that certain bacteria we need require meat in our diet, so he would advise against vegetarianism.

Previously mentioned, Professor Paul O'Toole, in studying how diet affects the microbiota of the aging population, has found that our gut microbiota is dominated by two types: Firmicutes and Bacteroidetes. The Western Diet, or the North American diet, is high in fat and protein. In this diet Bacteroidetes usually make up more than fifty-five percent of the gut microbiota, and sometimes, as much as eighty-percent. For a healthy microbiome, the reverse should be true. Historically, our ancestors ate a plant dominant diet and that is what our guts thrive on.[96]

Beyond variety, all the things we already know about a good diet apply to building a great garden of gut bacteria. A diet of healthy foods, preferably organic, some raw, some cooked, some meat, some fish, with the focus on lots of fresh vegetables will give you what you need. If you eat breads and cereals make them whole grain. Avoid processed foods, those with chemical additives, dyes, etc.

Fiber foods are particularly needed by the gut. Fiber (see the table below) is necessary to feed good bacteria. Healthy gut bacteria ferments fiber into short-chain fatty acids. By fiber, I don't mean bran flakes. There are specific prebiotic plants that have the kind of fiber gut bacteria thrive on. (See the section on prebiotics below) The consumption of these maintains the proper PH (acid/alkaline balance) of the large intestine at a range that supports the development of healthy bacteria.

Comparing Contemporary Diets, How They Affect the Microbiome

The basics of several popular contemporary diets:

> **Raw:** You eat only raw, uncooked vegetables and fruits, maybe some raw meat or fish.

Wahl's Protocol: Designed for autoimmune disease, nine cups of vegetables & fruit a day, raw or lightly cooked and exclude the major allergic foods: casein, soy, gluten.

Paleo: Eat like a caveman: vegetables, fruit, nuts, seeds, fish, meat, and eggs. Paleo excludes dairy, grain-based foods, legumes, extra sugar, refined fats, refined carbohydrates, processed foods.

Ketogenic: High protein, high fat, vegetables, no carbs, no sugars (including fruits)

Raw, Wahl's Protocol, Paleo, High Fiber, Low Carb, Gluten free, casein free, soy free diet, Ketogenic, etc., today, there are more diet plans available than you could try in a lifetime. Diet is a complex subject and I will not try to go into it in depth here. But, if you take a look at some of the diets most touted for good health, there are elements they all have in common.

1. The need for fiber—prebiotic food for good bacteria (High fiber, Raw, Paleo, Wahl's Protocol)
2. Enzymes from raw food to help break down food (Raw diet, Paleo diet, Wahl's Protocol)
3. Low sugar, low carb (or no sugar, no carb) to prevent overgrowth of yeast and bad bacteria (Ketogenic, Atkins diet, Anti-inflammatory diet.)
4. Avoidance of foods you may be allergic or sensitive to reduce inflammation in the gut. (Use an elimination diet to determine which foods you are sensitive to. Most frequent offenders are gluten, dairy and soy.)
5. Vitamin B for intrinsic factor- (organ meats, like liver, kidney, tongue and heart are rich in B vitamins.)

6. Vitamin D to enable calcium absorption and other gut functions.
7. Both meat and vegetables in diet, proportionally higher vegetables and lower sugar to increase Firmicutes and reduce Bacteroides. High numbers of Firmicutes bacteria are associated with obesity. (Wahl's Protocol, Raw, Paleo, High Fiber)
8. Added magnesium (unless you eat organic) to replace lack of minerals in foods produced in depleted soil.
9. Make sure your levels of zinc are normal. Zinc helps starve some bad bacteria.
10. Organic foods, if possible, to reduce pesticide and herbicide intake that kills bacteria.

If you feel worse on a high vegetable diet

Whenever you make a major change in your diet, you may feel worse, as bad bacteria dies off and new bacteria begins to replace it. If, however, that feeling continues for more than a week or two, oxalates may be a problem. Oxalates are naturally occurring substances found in certain otherwise healthy plant foods like spinach, rhubarb, swiss chard, okra, leeks, beets, sorrel and many others. They are part of the plants defense system. When consumed, oxalates form crystals in the body that act as irritants and can lead to kidney stones, joint problems, and many other disorders. In very large doses, such as sorrel soup, their intake can be fatal. See: https://sallyknorton.com/ for more information.) The only way to tell if this is a problem is to take high-oxalate foods out of your diet for several weeks and see what changes occur.

The FODMAPS Diet

The FODSMAPS diet (Fermentable Oligo-, Di-, Mono-saccharides And Polyols) has been helpful to many people. This diet cuts intake of specific foods that are broken down (fermented by bacteria in the large bowel) containing the following specific sugars:

- Oligosaccharides—"oligo" means "few" and "saccharide" means sugar. These molecules are made up of individual sugars joined together in a chain
- Disaccharides—"di" means two. This is a double sugar molecule
- Monosaccharides—"mono" means single. This is a single sugar molecule
- Polyols—these are sugar alcohols (however, they don't lead to intoxication!)

These sugars, and in particular, oligosaccharides, are prebiotic foods for bacteria. While designed to help digestive disease, it may be that elimination of these sugars reduces the population of "bad' bacteria. Or they may reduce gastric symptoms by eliminating difficult to digest foods. *Whether the FODSMAPS diet is good or bad for your microbiome is uncertain at this time. Long term elimination of Oligosaccharides may starve necessary bacteria as well as unhealthy bacteria.*

PREBIOTICS VERSUS PROBIOTICS

Many studies have demonstrated the beneficial effects of prebiotics and probiotics on our gut microbiota. Prebiotics are things that serve as food for beneficial bacteria and promote the growth of some "good" bacteria. Probiotics have live bacteria that can reproduce and help the microbiota keep its balance and diversity. The search is on right now for the best way to get good bacteria back into the intestines and colon, in the right balance, especially when the body is constantly under attack from antibiotics, antibacterials and other chemicals in our air water and food. While fecal microbiota transfer can accomplish that, it takes the right diet to sustain the new microbiome and keep it healthy. In a garden analogy, prebiotics are the fertilizer or plant food.

To use probiotics to improve your microbiome, you can take probiotic pills or consume fermented foods like yogurts, kefir milk and waters, and fermented vegetables (see below.) Homemade fermented foods were a part of our ancestor's diet from antiquity. When purchasing, you want the products with the most variety and quantity of live microorganisms available. In the garden analogy, probiotics are the seeds.

One important note about prebiotics, probiotics and fecal microbiota transplants

Prebiotics immediately before FMT is a good idea. You are providing your new microbiome with food it can use to survive in its new environment. **But probiotics is the addition of new bacteria- so do not take these while undergoing FMT.** You can take them to see if you can repair your microbiome and resolve your gut issues and if that does not help, then proceed with FMT. You can add probiotics a few weeks following your last FMT procedure after your transplant has had time to establish itself.

Prebiotics

Prebiotics are made up of non-digestible carbohydrates (fiber) that feed the bacteria in the microbiome. Naturally found in food, a prebiotic is not broken down or absorbed by the gastrointestinal tract. Instead, beneficial bacteria use this fiber as a food source in a process called fermentation. These are very specific types of fiber, not the psyllium or cereal fibers used as laxatives. Currently, there are three major types of prebiotics that are well documented: inulin, oligosaccharides and arabinogalactans. (See previous comments about FODSMAPS diet)

Prebiotics are considered functional foods in that they provide numerous health benefits and aid in the prevention and treatment of diseases and health conditions.

Examples of food sources that contain prebiotics are:

- Onions
- Leeks
- Radishes
- Carrots
- Coconut Meat & Flour
- Tomatoes
- Flax and Chia Seeds
- Bananas

- Garlic
- Chicory Root
- Jicama
- Dandelion Greens
- Yams
- Jerusalem Artichoke
- Asparagus

Probiotic Foods

Probiotic means "for life" and they do have important life-giving qualities. Probiotics are beneficial bacteria that keep you healthy and strong. With enough of them in your intestines, they can boost your immunity and help you digest foods.

In her book, *The Probiotic Promise, Simple Steps to Heal Your Body from the Inside Out,* (Da Capo, 2015) author, Michelle Schoffro Cook, MD, provides excellent information on probiotic foods. Some of it is included below.[97]

Yogurt: Yogurt is made from milk, either cow or goat. Bacteria is added to the milk and it is allowed to ferment. You can find it in all kinds of formats from sugar-laden "shots" to heavier Greek yogurt. Avoid high sugar yogurts as the sugar promotes growth of harmful yeasts. (See below for how to buy the best yogurt.) *Note: some people who are dairy sensitive can tolerate cheese and yogurt, but if that is not* *the case with you- then stay away from dairy. It is not worth the damage that inflammation from food sensitivities can cause.*

Cheese: Some cheeses offer probiotics, including: yogurt cheese (made from straining yogurt through a cheesecloth to thicken it) and some unpasteurized dairy-free cheeses made through the addition of probiotic cultures. These probiotic-rich cheeses usually contain the cultures used to inoculate them so the health benefits can vary widely depending on the probiotic powder or capsule contents used.

Cultured Butter: Butter is best when made from raw milk from cows who are grass fed. Butter can also be cultured (fermented) and it is an excellent and delicious way to get more probiotics into your diet. If you can, avoid butter that is pasteurized. You may be able to purchase raw, cultured butter in some health food stores, but most likely you are going to have to make it at home by using a culture starter you can order online.

Kefir: Yogurt and kefir is pasteurized before it comes to market, but then probiotic bacteria are re-introduced, so it's a probiotic food by the time it gets to you. Kefir is similar to a drinkable form of yogurt but is much healthier as it has many more strains of bacteria than yogurt does. It naturally contains B-vitamins that give an energy boost, aids digestion, and helps to regulate blood sugar and cholesterol levels. As with yogurt- avoid heavily sugared versions.

Kefir contains several major strains of friendly bacteria not commonly found in yogurt (e.g., Lactobacillus kefir, Leuconostoc mesenteroides, subsp. cremoris, and Lactococcus lactis subsp. diacetylactis).

Kefir also contains beneficial yeasts, such as Saccharomyces kefir, which can dominate, control and eliminate destructive pathogenic yeasts in your body. They protect the mucosal lining where unhealthy yeast and bacteria reside, forming a team that attacks and cleans up your intestines. Therefore, your body becomes more efficient in resisting such pathogens as E. coli and intestinal parasites.

The curd size of kefir is smaller than yogurt, making it easier to digest, which makes it a particularly excellent, nutritious food for babies, invalids and the elderly, as well as a remedy for digestive disorders.

Kimchi: Kimchi is a Korean dish made of fermented cabbage, chilis, and garlic. Research at Georgia State University found that the probiotics, namely L. plantarum, found in Korea's national food, confers protection against the flu by regulating the body's innate immunity.

Kombucha: Kombucha (pronounced kom-BOO-shuh) is a beverage that is believed to have been made in Russia and China for over 2000 years, although the exact origin is unknown. The bacteria and yeasts that form the kombucha culture form a type of "floating mat" on the surface of the black or green or other type of tea from which it is typically made. It improves immunity against some diseases. According to research, consumption of kombucha has potential for prevention of a broad-spectrum of metabolic and infectious disorders.

Some people have trouble with kombucha because they are sensitive to its airborne yeast, which is different from beneficial strains of yeast used in other probiotic drinks. Additionally, some kombucha teas can have too much sugar and will make your blood more acidic and elevate yeast and fungal infection.

Kvass: A Russian grain-based drink that is made by adding yeast to bread and water and allowing it to ferment, kvass in most health food stores is often made with beets or carrots instead. While carrot kvass has many of the same nutrients as carrot juice, it usually has much less sugar thanks to microbes that digest the sugar and confer probiotic benefits in the process. If you choose a beet-based kvass be sure to choose one that is non-genetically-modified since beets are usually GMO.

Miso: Miso is usually made from fermented soybeans although there are also rice and chickpea miso as well. A staple in the Japanese diet, miso is rich in vitamins, minerals, protein, good carbs, and probiotics (provided it isn't heated as it often is when used in miso soup). Regular consumption of miso has been linked to protection against cancer. A study published in the Hiroshima Journal of Medical Science found that the long-term consumption of miso on animals with lung cancer could exert cancer-preventive and protective effects. Be careful, as many people are allergic or sensitive to soy. It is very hard to digest.

Pickles or other fermented vegetables: Usually pasteurized. If sold at room temperature they do not have live probiotics. Look for a container labeled "live and active cultures" (or something similar) and sold in the refrigerator section. Few store-bought brands actually contain live probiotic bacteria, and the ones that do tend to advertise it, so you should be able to tell from reading the label. Fermented vegetables in brine (similar to sauerkraut) does lead to the development of beneficial bacteria and some yeasts that also boost health.

Sauerkraut: Sauerkraut is one of the most overlooked superfoods. Lactobacillus plantarum and L. mesenteroides found in this German staple actually fight off harmful infections like E. coli. L. plantarum has anti-viral effects making it a potentially ally treating colds, flu, ebola, HIV, chronic fatigue syndrome, or other viral conditions.

Probiotic Drinks: Look in health food stores and the natural aisle of your grocery store. These are drinks that are water, milk or vinegar based with flavorings added. Some are "sparkling water based." Many new ones are coming on the market. Look for low sugar products with a natural source of vitamins, minerals, amino acids and enzymes, along with beneficial bacteria (like Lactobacillus acidophilus and Lactobacillus delbreukii) and beneficial yeast (like Sacharomyces boulardii and Saccharomyces cerevisiae).

Vinegar: Look for raw or unpasteurized vinegar that mentions having the "mother." Vinegar that is unpasteurized will be cloudy. Hard to find in grocery stores—easier to find in health food stores.

Keep in mind that any probiotic-rich food needs to contain "live cultures" and be "unpasteurized." If a product does not have either of these claims on the label it is best avoided. Additionally, probiotic-rich foods need to be refrigerated. If you find them on the shelves in the center aisles of your grocery store that means the product has been pasteurized for preservation and no longer offers any of the benefits of live cultures.

To make these foods at home, you can buy live "starter" cultures from online sources such as:

www.yogurtathome.com/
www.culturesforhealth.com
www.etsy.com/shop/AnythingHealthyLLC

How to Buy Yogurt

One of the easiest sources of beneficial microbes is yogurt. But not all yogurts are created equal.

1. Look for yogurt that contains "live and active cultures". Some companies heat-treat yogurt after culturing it with the good bacteria, (killing both the good and bad bacteria) so it will last longer and reduce tartness. But to do you any good, the carton must say "live and active cultures." These live and active

bacteria promote gut health, boost immunity, and some believe may even be a key to becoming slim and trim.

2. Avoid any yogurt that lists sugar as the first ingredient. Using the grams of sugar listed on the label as a guide, a standard 5.3 oz. Individual container of yogurt should contain no more than 18 grams of sugar, and ideally less than 13 grams. Plain yogurt is the best choice. Try adding fruit, or a small amount of fruit juice sweetened jam or raw honey (not for babies), to plain strained yogurt just before you eat it. And, it is better to add the fruit or honey just before you eat it as opposed to it being pre-mixed. Be aware that between 6—9 grams of sugar actually occur naturally in a 6-ounce container of plain regular yogurt and more may come from the fruit itself. Heavy doses of sugar feed harmful bacteria and yeasts like Candida.

3. If you are buying it with fruit, make it real fruit. Yogurt should have real fruit instead of a mix of sugar and food coloring or vegetable juice. Make sure you see actual fruit listed as an ingredient, ideally before any added sugars.

4. Avoid artificial sugar substitutes. "Low sugar" varieties often are full of artificial sweeteners, especially aspartame or sucralose and they are not healthy substances.

5. Avoid thickeners. Some brands of yogurt cut costs by adding thickeners like gelatin, corn starch, milk protein concentrate, gums and pectin, rather than straining the yogurt to make it thick and creamy (which more than doubles the protein and lowers the lactose). These impostors are often labeled as "Greek style". Authentic Greek yogurt won't contain these thickening agents. Real Greek yogurt maintains 12-16 g protein per 5.3 to 6 oz serving or 19—23 g protein per 1 cup. Check the label and try to pick yogurt with the most protein and the least sugar.

6. Keep it simple. All that is needed to make yogurt is milk and live, active bacteria so plain yogurt should have nothing more.

Flavored yogurt can have more ingredients, but the list should be short and filled with words you can identify.

7. Is nonfat better? Not necessarily. If you are lactose sensitive—but can tolerate yogurt, the more fat the yogurt has the less lactose.

8. Milk sensitivity? Try goat yogurt. Yogurt made from long-eared goats (Nubian) is naturally sweeter than that from traditional goats. Redwood Hill Farms is a goat yogurt that tastes wonderful and alive.

KEFIR VERSUS YOGURT- WHICH HAS MORE CFU'S?

Colony forming units (CFU's) is the measurement you want to look for when judging probiotic foods and drinks. As an example of typical differences between kefir, yogurt and fermented vegetables:

Milk Kefir — 2.6 Billion Colony Forming Units per milliliter (CFU/ml);

Water Kefir — 1.2 Billion CFU/ml

Greek Yogurt — 60 Million CFU/gram (note for water, 1 milliliter = 1 gram)

Cabbage Sauerkraut — 5.3 Million CFU/gram

How to Buy Probiotic Supplements

There is a vast variety of these on the market. You will find most of them in vitamin or health food stores and online. Some are stable unrefrigerated but *most quality probiotic supplements need refrigeration* to keep the microbes alive and viable.

Some studies have found that only half of all probiotic products actually have the healthy bacteria listed on their labels. Many probiotic products are not prepared in a way that allows the most beneficial bacteria and yeast to thrive in your digestive system. Harsh stomach acids can kill probiotics, and if they do survive stomach acid they may not be the kind of probiotics that recolonize your inner ecosystem. Consumer Labs runs tests on probiotic supplements. (See: consumerlab.com/reviews/Probiotic_Supplements_and_Kefir/probiotics/)

CFU's or colony forming units, are measurements of the numbers of live bacteria in the supplement. There can be anywhere from one to 20 billion or even higher. The higher end of the scale is usually recommended for a person with severe diarrhea. But it's an individual number so I would say start low and work to higher numbers until you see how your body reacts. Adding probiotics may make you constipated or give you symptoms of bloating or gas. These can be signs that your body is detoxing.

Drink a lot of water to help your body flush out yeast, fungi or bacteria that may have been killed by the new bacteria introduced by the probiotics. If this is problematic, just back down to a lower CPU and give the new bacteria time for your body to adjust.

Quality is very important as these are highly perishable products. You want to know if they have been kept refrigerated at the store of purchase. Feel free to ask your store personnel about their practices- and if they know if they are delivered in refrigerated trucks. More reputable companies report the number of live organisms at the time of expiration as opposed to time of packaging.

Check the reputation of various brands. To see which brands of probiotics actually have what they claim on their labels, Consumer Labs has tested about forty of the top brands. See the website: consumerlabs.com.

Some strains are more likely to survive all the way to the gut, others are known to be too fragile. You can do an online search for this information if you are trying to get a specific strain.

Match strains to your needs. What problems do you have? Generally, more variety of strains is better and it is a good idea to mix Lactobacillius and Bifobacterium strains as they complement each other.

Check ingredients to see if yeast or molds were used to grow the probiotic. Some people are allergic to molds and react to foods created with molds as a base or additive.

Take them in the morning on an empty stomach or before bed. As mentioned previously, antibiotics and antimicrobials are meant to kill off bacteria- good or bad. *So, it is especially important to rebuild with probiotics or FMT following a course of antibiotics.*

Caution

Probiotic supplements *do* have an effect. Everyone's microbiome is different. Start slow, use high quality brands, increase amounts of cu's and variety gradually to see which ones your body likes. You may experience constipation or diarrhea from them. This is not necessarily a bad thing. Your body may go through a die-off as some bacteria species kill off others.

Now that you know how to care for your "gut garden" you may want to try a transplant. Getting the environment right before you add new bacteria from probiotics or fecal transplant will help ensure the success of the transplant.

CHAPTER TEN

Is FMT Right for You?

Do You Need FMT?

This section of the book is all about determining if dysbiosis (bacterial imbalance in the gut) is a part of your health issues and what you can do to change that. Before you start with probiotic supplements or get FMT treatments, you should try to define your diagnosis. Many people who will read this book will have already gone the route of traditional medical exams and tests without getting the answers they need.

If you have not already done so, **try to get a medical diagnosis of your condition:**

- Find the best gastroenterologist you can and have standard tests including colonoscopy and endoscopy. Also see a rheumatologist to see if you have an autoimmune condition that can be the cause of your condition.
- Do you have hidden food allergies that have not been addressed? Is your diet under control? Do you have leaky gut? Low stomach

acid is another very common perpetuating factor that affects people with chronic digestive illness. It is easy to treat and no amount of good bacteria will fix your gut if your digestive system is not working properly further up. Low stomach acid can be resolved with digestive enzymes. (When purchasing these makes sure they have been refined. Most are cultured on molds and if sensitive to molds you may react. Houston Enzymes, available online work for me.) These issues can sabotage the success of FMT. And, you may find, if you handle them correctly, that you may not need FMT treatment at all.

- If you have an infection such as C. diff, which has a ninety percent cure rate using FMT, you should definitely have FMT.

- If you have ulcerative colitis, cure rates in trials using FMT have had high rates of success, (when used five days a week over an eight week or more period of time) so it is a worthwhile treatment for UC and possible other similar conditions.[98,99,100,101]

- If you have an autoimmune disease, you can safely try FMT to see if it will help resolve symptoms. Look at chapter seven in this book for specific autoimmune conditions and the rates of success in trials using FMT.

- FMT specifically treats dysbiosis. Dysbiosis means an imbalance of normal intestinal flora and it may or may not be the underlying cause of your problem. If you respond well to probiotics then this is a clear indication that dysbiosis is a contributing factor in your illness. However, if you don't respond to probiotics this doesn't mean you won't benefit from FMT as probiotics are not as powerful and indeed can make your gut worse in the wrong proportions. Likewise, if your condition improves on antibiotics or when your gut is empty this also suggests dysbiosis is a problem.

Checking out Your Gut Bacteria

The best way to tell what the health of your gut is would be to test the quantity and variety of microbes in your gut. You can invest in a microbial diversity test to confirm that the problem is dysbiosis. However, interpretation of these tests is difficult unless you have a clinician or physician well-versed in bacteria to draw conclusions from them. These tests are available through your medical practitioner or direct from these sources:

- http://www.openbiome.org/(US)
- https://taymount.com/(UK)
- ubiome.com (USA)
- americangut.org (USA)
- my.microbes.eu (Europe)
- bioscreen.com (Australia)

WHO SHOULD NOT UNDERGO FMT

If you have history of bacteremia (a condition where the microbiota can get into the blood from an abrasion in the gut wall) or if you have had a perforated bowel or are at risk of a perforated bowel you may not be a good candidate for FMT.

If you have an anal fistula that is unresolved or if you have a temporary ileostomy, it is still possible to have FMT but you would want to have it done in a clinic as an added precaution.

Check out the "Frequently Asked Questions" on the Power of Poop website. To make an informed decision you must research the possible risks as well as the possible benefits.

Medications while on FMT Therapy

If you must be on antibiotics, FMT will not work for you. Antibiotics can be used prior to beginning FMT but must be stopped at least ten days before your transplant, as it kills bacteria, both good and bad. Used after FMT, it may kill off your new transplant and you will have to begin FMT again.

Autoimmune drugs: Again, as with antibiotics, this group of drugs will work against the newly transplanted bacteria.

Drugs that *seem* to not have any negative effects on the microbiome are: prednisone, Prilosec, Tylenol and Imodium. Particularly with patients who have ulcerative colitis or Crohn's disease, prednisone may be important to continue until there is no more bleeding or pain present.

Do not take aspirin or ibuprofen as they are destructive to your stomach lining and can increase bleeding.

If you are eating healthy foods that feed gut bacteria, have eliminated foods you are allergic or sensitive to, are staying away from microbials and antibiotics (except when absolutely necessary), avoiding environmental toxins, and getting good probiotics with live bacteria, you can make a big difference in your health, particularly if all this becomes a permanent lifestyle. But, if you are seriously ill with Crohn's Disease, colitis, or other autoimmune disease, have a long history of antibiotic treatment, or if you have or had a C. diff infection, then you will probably need something more intensive than diet to rebuild your microbiome.

The fastest and most certain way to establish colonies of good bacteria in your gut is through fecal microbiota transfer. When FMT is performed, you are taking live bacteria from a healthy gut and literally transplanting it. Transplanted via enema or colonoscopy, the bacteria does not have to make its way through the bodies gauntlet of acids, enzymes and bile. It is estimated that much of the probiotic bacteria we consume, whether in pill form or in foods, is destroyed long before it reaches the deeper parts of the intestines and finally, the colon. But when the fecal transplant is inserted directly into the colon via an enema, the microbes can be relatively safe there while they grow and multiply.

FMT in the USA

As previously discussed, you can get this treatment in the USA only if you have the diagnosis of C.diff and only after you have gone through three trials of antibiotics. *(see US provider list in the back of this book)* But you can go overseas, to England, Argentina, the Bahamas and other countries, *(see international provider list in back of this book)* to get treated for most conditions related to dysbiosis, including colitis, Crohn's Disease and some autoimmune conditions. Should those options be impossible, you can find and test a donor and perform fecal transplant yourself.

Providers Outside the United States

The **Taymount Clinic** in the U. K. is the premier FMT clinic in the world. Founder and Science Director, Glenn Taylor, virtually created the protocol and procedures now used by numerous practitioners throughout the United Kingdom, Europe and other countries. Glenn is a microbiologist with a background in engineering. Enid Taylor, ND, BSc, is Glenn's wife and clinic director. He says it was her work with food and digestion that inspired his research. He began to connect the health of our gut bacteria with both digestive and general health. He founded the clinic in 2003 with the objective of helping people with digestive health problems.

Along with their experienced staff, Glenn and Enid provide staff training and transplants for many other clinics in Europe and Canada. They will accept patients with dysbiosis and related conditions.

After much academic research and laboratory experimentation in harvesting, handling, refining and storing of the whole human microbiome, the directors tried implanting themselves with transplants from healthy, tested, individuals. They then conducted ongoing tests to measure the changes that occurred over time. They found that the new bacterial implants grew and were maintained in their new environments.

They continued to develop and refine safety protocols; including a three-month quarantine to ensure that all implants were healthy not only at time of collection but later, in case some dormant spore might develop. After extensive testing with themselves and staff, they had found a process that worked to not just solve an immediate health issue like C.diff., but one that would change the patients microbiome on a more permanent basis and include the complex variety of bacteria that cannot be found in any one probiotic formula. The three-month quarantine of frozen implants is not common to all clinics who perform FMT but is a good question to ask if considering other clinics.

Based on all of their research and experimentation and their history of having performed over 8,000 transplants they developed a standardized process for FMT.

As their website states, "as the research progresses, they are beginning to see exciting connections between the microflora and the immune system, which in their view is clearly highlighting the need for the medical and microbiological communities to join forces and concentrate more efforts into understanding the unique relationship between bacteria and the human immune system."

Sister locations are the **Institute of Predictive Personalized Medicine** in Bratislava, Slovakia and the **Taymount Clinic at the Bahamas Medical Center,** Nassau, Bahamas. My experience at the Taymount Clinic in the U.K. is described below.

In choosing an out of the country clinic, you will find a wide variety of process and treatment procedures. I can share with you my experience at Taymount, which was excellent. Their usual program consists of two weeks treatment and ten implants. You can also purchase implants to take home with you. The transplants are frozen and packaged in a way that gives you a window of 48 hours to get them to your home freezer. So, take that into consideration when making travel arrangements. You may also return to Taymount later if you need additional treatments. While flights overseas are expensive, lodging (using Air B and B) was reasonable and if you stay in the town where the clinic is located (and are able to walk) you may not require a car rental.

Taymount does not treat children under the age of sixteen. They will treat children ages 16-18 with parental consent. The Bahamas Clinic, on the other hand, has a pediatrician on staff who can treat children over the age of five.

My friend Allie went to the Bahamas for treatment and was also pleased. The **Bahamas Clinic** is attached to a medical facility with physicians on hand for consultation should you need that. People who have complications, (as did Allie with her anal fistulas and flares) may feel more secure if a doctor is on hand. The Bahamas, while a cheaper air flight was much more expensive in treatment costs (double the Taymount charge) and higher in lodging and car rental costs. Bahamas' traffic is tough but then, of course, there is the offset of the weather and beach access.

The Argentinian clinic, **Newbery Medicine**, located in Buenos Aires, was founded by Dr. Silvio Najt (1952—2016), a recognized leader in the development of FMT protocols in Argentina. Dr. Najt began his investigation into IBD in connection to his own child's illness. He studied Dr. Thomas Borody's work in Australia and with a team of medical specialist began treating people with FMT. He consulted with Glenn Taylor, founder of Taymount on many occasions. Their clinic can treat for a four-week period at a very reasonable cost.

Many of the out of U.S. providers listed in the back of this book will perform fecal transplants for many conditions including C.diff.

In the list, I have noted the ones that I know will definitely perform FMT for dysbiosis and other conditions. Providers in Canada and the USA can only use FMT as a treatment for C.diff. and then, only when antibiotics have failed.

MY EXPERIENCE AT THE TAYMOUNT CLINIC

When I decided to go to the Taymount clinic, friends asked why I would do that since I could continue with at-home procedures using my tested donor. My reasons to go to a clinic were many.

First of all, I might be missing something in my self-treatment and could learn more than I already knew about the whole process. Second, I would be getting transplants from multiple donors, receiving more varied samples of bacteria. My personal history included years of antibiotics and later, years of antifungals. My age (68) was also a factor. I knew that the aging process tended to reduce your microbiomes vitality and a more intensive therapy might be necessary. Third, I wanted this book to reflect as much current information as possible and being at the clinic would allow me to speak directly with the clinic directors and staff as well as patients.

The thought that I might be able to correct the damage done and replace the bacteria I had lost through those years of inappropriate treatment was exciting. I knew my digestive system was not functioning properly and I still had occasional bouts of systemic candida, a whole-body yeast infection that caused break out rashes, stomach issues and difficulty focusing when the infection was in full gear. I also had severe gluten intolerance and diagnosis of diverticulosis. I had cysts on my pancreas and liver and sometimes an elevated pancreatic tumor marker. My stool was pale yellow, an indicator of something wrong with the gall bladder or liver. In addition, my father and brother both had colon cancer and my mother breast cancer. It seemed reasonable that a healthy microbiome (and immune system) might help solve some of those issues and perhaps help prevent those cancers.

There were two clinics I was aware of that provided fecal transplants for those with digestive conditions other than C.diff. infections. They were the Taymount Clinic in England and the Bahamas Medical Center Fecal Transplant Clinic, (now there are several more- see list of providers in appendix.) I decided on Taymount. The cost of treatment at Taymount was half that of the Bahamas Clinic. Because of this and because the Taymount people had established a therapeutic model, had trained the staff at the Bahamas Clinic and seemed to me to be the top experts internationally in this field, I chose Taymount.

So, after multiple conversations, and more research, I booked two weeks of treatments at Taymount and bought a plane ticket to London. I also got an Airbnb-shared apartment in Hitchin, a town twenty minutes away from the clinic site which is located in Letchworth Gardens.

In the weeks before you go to the clinic you are required to do one or two water colonics . (A water colonic is the flushing out of the bowels using gentle water pressure. Water colonic machines were at one time used in most gastrointestinal doctor's offices but are now found at spas and wellness centers. Much preferable to using a harsh chemical clean-out.) So, I had one water colonic done in the states prior to leaving.

Then I was on my way to England, by myself. At present, new patients at the clinic undergo two weeks of five treatments per week. Once you have been a patient there you can come back for "topping off" treatments of shorter duration. Clinic co-director Edith Taylor says that spaced out treatments might be more beneficial but that so many people travel long distances to get there they do the intensive two-week therapy. They also will not perform less than two weeks (ten transplants) for new patients, as they feel you need that minimum to see results especially if you have a severe or chronic condition.

On the plane people chatted. My seatmate wanted to know where I was going. She, like many people I had talked with recently, wanted to know why I was going to England. Am I going alone? Is it a vacation? If not- then what? So, I reluctantly told her I was going to have a medical procedure done there. Really? Because it is cheaper? Because....why.? The unspoken question is what kind of medical procedure? I was not about to get into a public discussion of my bowel problems. So, as I did with some of my friends back home, I hedged and dodged the questions.

Arriving at Heathrow airport from the states, I was tired. But I jumped immediately into a rental car, got my head wrapped around the "drive on the left" thing, dealt with roundabouts and adapted to a new car. If you go, I highly recommend getting an in-car navigator from the car rental agency. It was well worth the price. Without its calm English voice continually giving me directions, I would never have made it to Hitchin. Hitchin is a lovely ancient town about twenty-five minutes away from the clinic. The clinic is located in the commercial district of the more contemporary town of Lechworth Gardens. If I were to do it again, I would exchange charm for convenience and stay closer to the clinic.

In my B&B I did a final clean out prep with magnesium citrate powder mixed with water. That is what I use in the US for colonoscopy prep. I was grateful that my Airbnb hostess was not at home that day.

The clinic was located in an old building remodeled and redecorated nicely in a traditional English style. I was welcomed by Dawn, the office manager, and seated in a nice reception area, with an extremely clean, modern bathroom (thank goodness) close by.

There was no interview that day, no telling of my story to anyone. That had all been done via email and phone prior to my arrival date. If you are expecting a personal consultation, you may need to ask beforehand if that can be scheduled. It is not a part of the treatment per se. Once there, the focus is totally on treatment not on your history.

While waiting for my first appointment, I met other patients. There was Robert (not his real name) who looked like a well to do, middle-aged businessman. He had traveled all the way from New Zealand for treatment and it was his second time. He believes the first treatments helped him and he wants more. He is here for "digestive issues," I did not want to press him for details. Then there was Peter from Denmark (not his real name.) Blond and handsome with a great smile. He looked the picture of health. He said he was once one of the top national wrestling champs in Denmark but has stomach issues and has lost a great deal of muscle. He is not getting nutrition from his food.

Lucy, who was my therapist while I was there, greeted me with enthusiasm. She explained to me that she had been doing colonics commercially for six years before working at Taymount. She tried colonics initially as a way to deal with her own health issues and then began performing them for others. As I talked with them, most of the therapists and both directors explained that they became interested in this field in an attempt to help their own or a family member's health issues. Most have had the treatment themselves.

Lucy got right down to business. "Go in the bathroom, empty your bladder, take off your clothes except your bra and put on the hospital gown in case of an accident." I asked for the heat to be turned up. The British love the cold. She said, "first we are doing a colon cleansing." I explained that, as I had been instructed, I had done a water colonic in the states before leaving as well as a "prep" in the apartment two days before. She explained that another would be necessary because it was so important for the new bacteria to have a clean surface to grow on.

I am stunned to see what is still left in my colon after all the prep I did. When the colonic treatment is finally completed, I go to the toilet to empty out what may be left. After that, it's "lie down on the table."

Lucy gently puts some Vaseline up my butt and here we go. No more chit chat till the job is in progress. A plastic tube, very small diameter, thank God, sliding in. "Take a deep breath, now let it out slowly." Gently, she eases it in. The tubing goes inside you at a depth of about six inches. That is deeper than my Fleet enema bottle can go. They say that extra depth is important. "Are you ok?" she asks repeatedly. "Ok, now I am going to put the implant in," Lucy says. She uses a plastic syringe to pull the implant material from a cup and then connects the syringe to the tubing. I felt a cool liquid coming into me. Not warm, cool. She said, "Now I am adding saline solution." Here, she used a different plastic syringe with water/saline solution in it. She attached this to the tube still inside me and "flushed" the tubing clean. "Deep breath, let it out." Then she took out the thin plastic tube and it was all over. No discomfort whatsoever.

Next, you lie on your left side, your back, your right side, with the table tilted so that your head is down, enlisting gravity to help keep the implant inside as long as possible. For me, some days that was four hours, but most days it was only as long as I was lying on the table. Once I got up, I had to quickly go to the toilet. While this was disappointing, Lucy kept reassuring me, saying that it was helping even if inside you for just 30 minutes. Lucy then gave me a prebiotic powder called Bimuno which I am supposed to take very small doses of each day to feed the new bacteria. Prebiotic powder, (perhaps one quarter of a teaspoon) is also mixed in with the transplant material and some saline solution before the procedure. (FYI, side effect of Bimuno is gas.)

Everyone that came to the clinic during my time there, was eager to talk about their condition with the staff and directors. From a time element, that would be impossible, so the directors meet with patients in a group setting once a week. That is even better as the patients can share information among themselves, as well as hearing from the staff. It's a great opportunity for an exchange of knowledge and experience.

On the day, I met with the clinic directors, there were nine patients waiting to speak with directors Glenn and Enid Taylor. There were people from all over the world. In addition to Peter and Robert, who I had already met, there was a mother from the United States with her son. They both had recurrent Candida problems. An older woman, pleasant and outgoing from Manchester, UK, had come in the hopes of getting help for her grandchildren. A woman with either Parkinson's disease or multiple sclerosis who could not speak and barely walk, was supported by her husband. A man in his thirties also from England, had been given five antibiotics in one day in the hospital and had a massive reaction. He had gone into cardiac arrest and was in intensive care for several weeks. He was released but suffering from vasculitis, severe neuropathy, with needles and pins sensation in his feet and legs so intense he could barely walk. He was hoping FMT might help him. There was a quiet young man from Norway with severe ulcerative colitis.

Some of the things I learned that day:
The only probiotic the clinic recommended (at that time) was Symprove, (http://www.symprove.com/) a truly disgusting tasting liquid with the smell of vomit to it- but they say it is able to make it through the stomach acid and all the way to the colon. Symprove is available in Europe and can be shipped to the US.

Glenn Taylor, Founder and Co-Director of the clinic said in regard to probiotic foods like yogurt, they must have live organisms without added sugars. Sweetened yogurts are not helpful. He said take a probiotic pill on an empty stomach first thing in the morning for maximum value.

When asked if donor diet matters, he said: "Absolutely. Our donors are coached to eat the best organic diet, high in fruits and vegetables and pasture-fed animal products. They eat high fiber and natural sources of probiotics, as in kefir and probiotic yogurts on a regular basis."

He stresses that without the right diet, the beneficial bacteria cannot thrive. "The microbiome is like the most varied pet shop in the world; if you bought a pet, you would ensure that you were feeding it properly." The same goes for the gut microflora, which individually thrive on particular food groups; absence of these food groups results in the absence of a bacterial group. "Along with the diet, it is important that the donor does not smoke—all the pathogenic smoking debris gets transferred into the swallowed mucus and ends up in the digestive tract to be excreted in the feces. We would also not use a donor who drank a lot of alcohol for obvious reasons."

If you get **digestive enzymes** they should be special brands, Taymount sells one. Digestive enzymes are grown on molds. You can have a reaction to the molds, which I do, (vertigo and headache) unless they have been highly refined. In my personal experience, I react allergically to most digestive enzymes while Houston Digestive enzymes (due to a special refining process that removes all traces of mold) are fine. I find that they help cut the sugar cravings I have after eating a meal.

Since I have a grandchild with **autism**, I was particularly interested in what they might have observed with patients who had autism as well as a digestive disease. Taymount treats only adults. But when adults on the autism spectrum came there for digestive issues, families began reporting back that the patient was suddenly making eye contact and responding socially as they had never done before. Not cures, but specific improvements. He said, as a result, the Bahamas clinic, which is attached to a hospital with physicians and pediatrician on staff, began to accept young adults and teens with autism. They reported similar experiences. In fact, one autistic child treated at the Bahamas Clinic began to speak after treatment. Taylor says that, in addition to the mother's bacteria, the microbiome of the people who first *deliver and touch* the baby—gets transmitted to the infant.

When asked what he thought the connection was between autism and gut microbes, Taylor said that **Clostridia bacteria**, when allowed to overgrow, produce neurotoxins. When a child is put on antibiotics that wipe out good bacteria, that overgrowth can occur as a result. Conversely, when a child is put on a heavy antibiotic like Vancomycin, it temporarily reduces the Clostridia and autism symptoms can disappear only to come back once the child is off the antibiotic.

In discussing the implants, Taylor stressed that they are not fecal transplants but bacterial transplants. Taymount has developed a complex process of extracting the bacteria from the material not just straining it. Hormones and toxic materials are filtered out and it is twice centrifuged *cold*, as heat can destroy it. The transplants should not be exposed to oxygen. The bacteria is put into a nitrogen environment immediately. From each donation, they wind up with a thirty-milliliter quantity and freeze it immediately. When it is defrosted for use, they feed it with small amounts of prebiotics, (Bimuno.) No fresh stool is used. All transplants are frozen and quarantined for three months. Every implant used for a patient has a spare small sample in their freezer forever, labeled with donor and recipient, so they can trace back any problems. The clinic's biggest problem is their increasing need for freezer storage space. Currently, they have thirty different donors, each providing unique stool due to their lifestyle and diet.

Patients report that, in addition to their digestive problems solved, these symptoms were reported improved or eliminated: attention deficit, depression, symptoms of multiple sclerosis, Parkinson's Disease, hand tremors and uveitis. Taylor remarked that *the one branch of medicine that seemed to understand the far-reaching effects of the microbiome were the immunologists.*

Taylor says, "You need meat to feed some kinds of bacteria. I've seen too many sick vegetarians." Variety in the foods you eat is key. He said use a chart to see if you are eating fifty different foods a week. (I tried it-it's not hard to do.) He recommends the book, *Diet Myth* by Tim Spector.

Regarding the stomach, Taylor adds that chlorine in water is not so much a problem as stomach acid is harsher. If you use proton pump inhibitors (for GERD and acid reflux) you will lose intrinsic factor needed to get Vitamin B. Vitamin B deficiency and folate deficiency can cause dementia.

At the time I was there, the Taymount staff were in the process of training staff for several new clinics in Europe. Clinics are opening in Germany, Canada, Cypress, Slovakia, and Spain in the future. Also, Dove Clinic in England will be performing transplants. They do not own other clinics but provide the licensed method of FMT, train their staff and sell the implants. (See the provider list in the appendix.)

The clinic now offers a service. You can donate your own stool and they will keep it stored and implant you with it in future if you have to take a course of antibiotics. And, you can also have your own fecal bacteria tested by Taymount to have an accurate measurement of the quality and quantity of your own microbiome.

They tell people at the clinic to watch for changes—but warn you that it takes about three months to build a new microbiome. They will contact you three months after treatment to ask if you have seen any changes.

It's now ten months from the time I was treated at the Taymount clinic. What changes have I seen? My pancreatic tumor marker is normal. My stool has gone from pale, sickly yellow to a robust brown. Unlike when I did this at home, it has retained that color consistently for ten months. My immune system is strong — no colds or flu or strep despite contact with relatives and friends with the same. I have had strep, colds and conjunctivitis each winter for as long as I can remember. This winter, despite contact with many others who were sick, I remained healthy. That is remarkable.

Other changes I would like to see? Slight tremor in left arm is still there. Bowel is stable, no diarrhea, unless I inadvertently eat some gluten or wheat. I am very happy about the stool color change, the tumor marker and the apparent improvement in immune function. Was it worth it? Absolutely, especially because I believe that my sons, grandchildren, and daughter in law may someday benefit from my experience.

CHAPTER ELEVEN

Do It Yourself Fecal Transplant

Disclaimer

These fecal transplant at home instructions are based on the author's experiences and experiences of others. They are not medical advice. FMT is still considered an experimental procedure without known future consequences. Discuss your options with your doctor before doing fecal microbiota transplant (FMT). It is critical that your donor be tested properly before FMT and that all directions about handling of the material be followed. An outwardly healthy person could carry an a parasite or blood borne illness that might not be obvious or known by that person.

Introduction

If you follow all of these instructions carefully, you should have no problem performing your own fecal transplants. However, it is always helpful to have medical supervision, especially as you go through the testing phase. Even if your doctor cannot perform a transplant due to government or medical regulations, he may still be able to give you guidance in the process. If you are having a transplant due to a C. diff infection, he may be able to actually perform the transplant. At the very least, he may be able to order tests for you or your donor that will save you money if you (or your donor's) insurance covers them. See the list of practitioners in the previous chapter. The Power of Poop website (thepowerofpoop.com) and the Fecal Transplant Foundation (thefecaltransplantfoundation.org) association websites also have provider lists.

The First Step - Finding a Donor

This is the most important part of fecal transplant. **Do not under any circumstances, skip the donor testing process.** Even if you know the person well, you (and they) may not know what they have been exposed to in the past. In addition to my instructions below, you should check the Power of Poop website (powerofpoop.com) for additional, detailed instructions on finding and testing donors.

Start with the people you know best. Think in terms of current friends, relatives and people from your past who know you well. If you have known them for at least six months that is helpful, but the longer the better. Ideally, they would be healthy, fit, have no gastrointestinal problems and eat a reasonably healthy diet. They should not be obese as there is some evidence that a tendency to gain weight (or lose weight) can depend on whose microbiota you use.

If you can pick someone to approach who already has a healthy lifestyle and has an open mind about alternative medicine, you will be way ahead of the game. I don't mean to say that FMT is alternative medicine because it was well on its way to becoming mainstream until the FDA made it almost impossible for the average gastroenterologist to use as a therapy. And it is the gold standard for C. diff infections that don't respond to antibiotics.

You will need to be able to sound credible, showing articles and books about FMT and first-person stories of those who have benefitted from it. There are certainly enough scholarly articles online to show what positive results it has had in clinical trials. You will also need to show how much you need it. People who become donors will also be concerned about liability issues and you may offer them something in writing to relieve them of that concern. A disclaimer would say that you, the donee, knows what you are doing and take full responsibility for any negative outcome.

When asking, try to introduce the topic in as scientific and logical way possible. Show them credible articles on the topic. For example, in Massachusetts, the company OpenBiome, pays for donated stool, freezes it, stores it and sells it to hospitals and medical practitioners all over the country. They have shipped (at writing time of this book) over 20,000 transplants, used by 800 practitioners in forty US states. This is a valid medical practice that has been around for a while. You can show them the history and explain that in other countries, this procedure is legal for your condition and is helping hundreds of people each year. You can show them the first person reports on the Taymount Clinic site and Power of Poop sites. You can share this book with them.

A family member or friend is easiest to approach. But if that fails, you can also find people who are charitable or kind, who just want to help out other people. As seen on the POP website, one New Yorker placed an ad in a periodical requesting help and got forty-five replies. She was able to select an appropriate donor from these and successfully performed her transplant. So, it is not impossible to find someone even if your nearest and dearest can't or won't qualify. Don't let fear of rejection stop you from improving your health.

If you know someone, their history and their past and present relationships, you will be aware of what countries they have been in, who they have been spending time with, etc. See the "donor exclusion" items below. Ask these questions without being offensive. Or, you can type them into a form with yes or no answers. A printed-out form, (see appendix) may be more comfortable for you both when asking these very personal questions. Your donor will have to agree to one or two blood draws and, of course, be willing to provide a fecal sample.

As explained on the Power of Poop website, an email may be the best way to make the request. This gives you the chance to word your request perfectly and it gives the person time to look at your message, look at supporting information you may supply, research it and really think about it before responding.

From POP's website are these points to cover in your request:

- I need to ask you a favor as I'm in a bad way.
- This is what has been happening to me over the past X years.
- The only hope left to me is an unusual treatment, a fecal transplant.
- A fecal transplant works in a similar way to a blood transplant or a bone marrow transplant only less invasive.
- The idea is for the infusion of 'good bugs' to conquer the 'bad bugs' and gradually restore good health.
- This treatment is not yet mainstream but is gaining acceptance in the medical community as more studies are done and success rates proven.
- I am looking for a donor and am hoping that you can help.
- There is some pre-testing involved, but no cost to you.
- Here are some articles/links that will give you more information about the procedure.
- Here are two donor stories telling why they decided to help. (Get these from POP's website)
- Even better, refer them to a person who has had this procedure or pay (an office visit) for them to speak with a supportive physician.

- I totally understand if you are not comfortable with the idea, but if you can't help I would greatly appreciate if you could think of someone else who might.
- What do you think?
- Include any supporting information, websites or articles on the topic.

Testing is Critical!

The Infectious Diseases Society of America has created a basic guide for practitioners to use in the donor screening process as seen here:

Infectious Diseases Society of America Consensus Guidance
on Donor Screening and Stool Testing for FMT
(See: http://www.idsociety.org/FMT/)

> *"Preferred donor is an intimate, long-time partner of adult patient or, in the case of a pediatric patient, an adult first-degree relative, close family friend, or well-screened universal donor."*

You may want to be careful in using a mother as donor for her own child. If the child has significant bacterial issues, the mother may have passed them onto the child at birth as maternal bacteria is given to the child as he or she passes through the birth canal. However, if the mother has no history of antibiotic use and no history of any gastric issues, then she might be acceptable as a donor.

> *"For the purposes of informed consent, donors should be over the age of 18. However, children could also potentially serve as donors as long as both parental consent and child assent (i.e., agreement to serve as a donor) are obtained."*

"Donor questionnaire should be similar to current protocols for screening blood donors, see AABB Donor History Questionnaire Documents available at: http://www.fda.gov/BiologicsBloodVaccines/BloodBlood Products/ApprovedProducts/LicensedProductsBLAs/ BloodDonorScreening/ucm164185.htm)"

This questionnaire is designed for blood donors not for fecal transplants. Many of the questions do not relate at all to FMT procedures. And the intensive screening of blood through lab tests should cover all the known pathogens to look for in bacterial transfer. But some of the questions and answers may give you an idea of possible problem areas.

The other concern would be that a person is asymptomatic at the time of testing. At the Taymount clinic, all donations are held for three months (frozen) before use to make sure the donor does not come down with some undetected illness that did not show up in testing. But, if you want to use fresh stool- then you would observe the donor for three months and then test them. Or you can test your donor, then take the donated stool, freeze it (according to directions in this book or the POP website) and then hold it for three months to see if any symptoms show up in your donor. After the three months quarantine period, you can proceed with testing the stool. When the test results come back positive you can proceed with the transplant. It is your choice.

Below are questions that are important to ask. These things would *not* show up on the required blood or fecal tests.

Donor exclusion criteria should include:

- Obesity (As mentioned before, there is evidence that obesity affects gut microbes in a negative way and that it may be possible to transfer the tendency to be obese to the donee, if the donor is overweight.)

- Infectious disease, including exposure to HIV or Hepatitis.
- History of risky sexual activity, drug use, or had recent tattooing or piercings. (if you would like to put these questions to your donor in an impersonal form, you can print out and use the list of questions for potential blood donors at: http://www.fda.gov/BiologicsBloodVaccines/BloodBloodProducts/ApprovedProducts/LicensedProductsBLAs/BloodDonorScreening/ucm164185.htm)
- A history of antibiotic treatment during the preceding three months of donation. (It may be more appropriate to ask if they have_ever been on an extended course of antibiotics.)
- A history of intrinsic gastrointestinal illnesses, including inflammatory bowel disease, irritable bowel syndrome, gastrointestinal malignancies or major gastrointestinal surgical procedures.
- You want to ask about episodes of diarrhea, constipation, stomach pain, use of anti-acids, proton pump inhibitors. These can be indications of undiagnosed bowel disorders.
- A history of autoimmune or atopic illnesses or ongoing immune modulating therapy. (These can include the well-known diseases like Type I and Type II diabetes, lupus, multiple sclerosis, Parkinson's Disease, rheumatoid arthritis, celiac disease, Sjögren's Syndrome, ankylosing spondylitis, alopecia areata, vasculitis, temporal arteritis and psoriasis. I would also include persons with multiple chemical sensitivities and multiple allergies to this exclusion list.)
- A history of chronic pain syndromes (fibromyalgia, chronic fatigue) or neurologic, neurodevelopmental disorders, Metabolic syndrome, obesity (BMI of >30), or moderate-to-severe undernutrition (malnutrition)

- A history of malignant illnesses or ongoing oncologic therapy. (This includes a history of chemotherapy or radiation therapy.)

Other Concerns About Donors:

Age may make a difference as the microbiome diminishes in older persons, and it is believed, not fully developed until a child is about age three. Older than ten and younger than fifty is a good rule of thumb, although the health of the person is a more important factor than their age. There may be, as yet unknown, elements of compatibility issues between donors, so if you see no change from one donation, don't give up. Another donor may make the difference. Pregnant donors are not ideal as research has shown that the microbiota change during pregnancy. Also, estrogen is a risk factor for both gut illness and autoimmune illness, which is why autoimmune illness can be triggered or go into remission, during pregnancy. For the same reason, it may be best not to use a donor who is on birth control medication. Male donors are somewhat preferred over female donors if you have the choice.

The Tests You Need

If you have gone over the above questions and asked about all the exclusion factors above, and you are satisfied your potential donor is a good candidate, you can proceed to testing.

There are two kinds of testing. The first is blood tests where your donor will go to a local lab, have blood drawn and the blood will be sent away for testing. It may take two weeks or more to get back results depending on which lab you are using. You may be able to get many of these tests done for free (especially the sexually transmitted disease tests) at your local health department or a clinic. You may have to go to a separate clinic for some of the tests.

The second part are fecal tests that check for parasites. In this case you will pick up or be sent via mail, a fecal test kit or kits. You will need a good amount of fecal material (one whole bowel movement) from your donor to fill up vials in the test kits. When you get this sample, check it against the Bristol Stool Chart (see the appendix or https://en.wikipedia.org/wiki/Bristol_stool_scale) so you know what healthy stool looks like. If your sample does not look healthy, wait a week and ask your donor for another. If the second one looks poor, you may not want to use this donor.

Follow the directions carefully and fill vials to proper levels. Make sure all identifying info is readable. Send these off.

Minimum Tests for FMT Donors

Serum (Blood)Testing (to be performed within 4 weeks of donation):

- HAV-IgM - Clinical: Hepatitis A IgM Antibody, Serum
- HBsAg - HBsAg is the surface antigen of the hepatitis B virus. It indicates current hepatitis B infection.
- Anti-HCV-Ab - The Hepatitis C Antibody Test
- HIV-EIA - Screening test for HIV
- RPR - Screening test for syphilis

NOTE: Your local health department may test your donor for basic sexually transmitted diseases such as syphilis, gonorrhea, and chlamydia and HIV for free.

More information on this topic can be found at: http://www.fda.gov/BiologicsBloodVaccines/BloodBloodProducts/ApprovedProducts/LicensedProductsBLAs/BloodDonorScreening/ucm164185.htm) Then enter "blood donor screening" in the search engine.

Stool Testing (to be performed within 4 weeks of donation):

- C. difficile toxin B (preferably by polymerase chain reaction or PCR)
- Culture for enteric pathogens (bad bacteria)
- O+P, if travel history suggests (ova and parasite)

Your doctor (or your donor's doctor) may be able to help you with the tests by ordering them for you or your donor.

Direct to Patient Tests

These are lab companies that don't require you to go through your doctor. You can order these tests yourself and get the results mailed to you.

Direct Labs

Direct Labs offer a wide variety of functional medicine tests through laboratories including BioHealth, Metametrix, Doctor's Data, Genova Diagnostics, ELISA/Act Biotechnologies & ImmunoLabs. They do NOT offer blood tests for customers outside the USA, however all fecal, urine & hair tests are available for international customers.

For people who want to test their donor (or themselves) without having to go through their doctor or insurance, use the following tests from Direct Labs:

- CDSA 2.0 w/Parasitology-Genova Kit
- Clostridium Difficile: Colitis Toxins A & B-BioHealth Kit
- Cryptosporidium Antigen-BioHealth Kit
- GI Effects Gastrointestinal Function Comprehensive Profile (One Day Collection)-Genova Kit

Other lab options if you have a physician's order:

- LabTesting Direct (USA)
- True Health Labs (USA)
- My Med Labs (USA)
- Great Plains Laboratory (USA)
- Cyrex Labs (USA)
- Private BloodTests (UK)

Labs for Fecal Diversity Tests Only

If you want to make sure your donor has a wide variety of healthy bacteria- you can now get that tested at one of the following companies.

- Open Biome (USA)
- uBiome (USA)
- American Gut (US)
- Taymount Clinic (UK)
- MyMicrobes (Europe)
- Bioscreen (Australia)

Additional Tests

Most FMT clinics recommend additional testing above the minimal requirements. Here are some links explaining other recommendations for tests that can keep FMT experience safe and productive according the following organizations:

- Openbiome: http://www.openbiome.org/safety/
- John Hopkins (USA): http://www.hopkinsmedicine.org/gastro-enterology_hepatology/clinical_services/advanced_endoscopy/fecal_transplantation.html
- Taymount Clinic brochure (UK): https://taymount.com/patients/faq

- Newbery Clinic (Argentina): http://newberymedicine.com
- Centre for Digestive Diseases (Australia): http://www.cdd.com.au

If you click on some of the organizations and clinics listed above you will see that there are a variety of tests and beliefs about what constitutes safe donor testing. Some of these tests are adjusted by location, given that certain pathogens are more common in specific regions. But most of them are standard and are chosen to keep patients safe from known pathogens.

How to Interpret Your Results

Ask your physician to help interpret your test results. In addition, you can access these resources below. Also, see the Power of Poop website for more information on this subject.

- How to interpret a Genova Comprehensive Digestive Stool Analysis
- How to interpret Metametrix GI Effects stool profile
- How to interpret a Doctors Data Comprehensive Stool Analysis & Parasitology (Video)

You can order these tests through Direct Labs

CHAPTER TWELVE

Preparation

Decisions

There are several options with the various aspects of the FMT procedure. Go through these options to decide for yourself which will work best for your particular health situation and comfort level.

Decide if you are going to use antibiotics to kill off bad bugs prior to FMT.

This is not mandatory, opinions differ. Many people who have overgrowths of bacteria such as C.diff and Klebseilla pneumonia have used antibiotics first with good results. Those who are experiencing overgrowth due to overuse of antibiotics often don't want to risk another round. This is between you and your doctor to determine the best course of action prior to FMT. (*Note: children and adults with autism may benefit from a round of antibiotics such as Vancomycin to kill off the existing bad bacteria. Clinical trials of FMT for autistic individuals often precede transplants with this antibiotic. Discuss with your doctor.*) If you do use antibiotics, you want them completely out of your system at the time of transplant or you will risk killing off your new bacteria. Each antibiotic has its own life span. Check on this, and if you are taking antibiotics for any reason, stop them *at least* a week before your transplant.

Decide if you will be freezing your implant and how to freeze it.

Frozen FMT allows you the flexibility that a donor doesn't. Some believe it does not have the same quality as fresh as the bacteria is compromised by freezing in home refrigerators, (unless flash frozen with dry ice first.) All the professional clinics flash freeze their implants prior to using.

Each time I received a donation, I cut it into two portions, freezing one and using the other one that day. Take the fresh material, add a few drops of glycerin, put it into a Ziploc bag, seal the bag, mash the bag with your fingers to mix it up. (Do not use more than a few drops per sample as glycerin can act as a laxative.) Then immediately flash freeze it with dry ice (see below) then put the frozen material into your home freezer. (Never put the dry ice in your freezer.) The liquid glycerin has been shown to keep the bacterial cell walls from bursting during the freezing process. Without glycerin, you will lose species. To maximize the potency of the FMT it is best to freeze the sample without adding water. The more interference (air and water) the more the potency is compromised.

Dry Ice Cautions

While I believe that the flash freeze method preserves the bacteria better than just putting it in your home freezer, there are issues using the dry ice.

Freezing in commercial labs is different from freezing at home. Labs that store FMT, quick freeze it and store it at minus 20 degrees Fahrenheit. Home freezers are around 0 degrees Fahrenheit. You can use dry ice which is **minus 109 degrees (!)** Fahrenheit but there are several concerns with this.

First there are safety issues. Especially if you have children- you may not want to risk their exposure to dry ice. It can burn your skin on touch. As it melts, it gives off toxic carbon dioxide gas. It cannot be stored in a refrigerator as it will break the temperature gauges and freeze whatever is around it. You cannot store it in an airtight container as it may explode. In my own case, I used the dry ice only to quickly freeze the stool and then later put the transplants in my regular freezer. When finished with it, place the dry ice in a place where it can melt safely and no pets or children can access it.

Some people will freeze stool so they can have a quarantine period before use. That three-month period would ensure that your donor did not pick up a bug between the time they were tested and the time of donation. (During those three months you can observe the donor and check on his health.) It also gives you the option of performing the transplant whenever it is convenient for you.

The amount of frozen FMT you use will depend on how much you have and when you will next see your donor. There are no hard and fast rules.

Using previously frozen FMT

It should take an implant or stool donation about two hours at room temperature to defrost. If after the two hours, it still is frozen, you can put the Ziploc bag or implant container in a cup of tepid (room temperature but never hot!) water. The end mix will be a comfortable temperature to have inside you, but not so hot that the good bacteria are killed. If it is too cold, it will tend to run out of you. Once it's defrosted, prepare the stool per directions below.

How long can you store it if frozen?

We don't yet know how long frozen stool can be kept. OpenBiome states that although further research has yet to be done "microbiological culturing experience suggests that samples may be stored for up to 6 months at -20°C without a significant loss of viability." The Taymount Clinic suggests using implants up to six months old if kept frozen.

Decide what kind of "Clean-Out" you will do if this is your first FMT:

By all means do a clean-out before your *first* transplant. The idea is that the new bacteria cannot adhere to intestinal walls that have old, dried fecal matter lining them. *Even if you have had diarrhea for years- this condition may still exist.* Give your new bacteria a nice clean surface to adhere to. Very important per the Taymount Clinic instructions. So much so, that two water colonic treatments are required before they will perform an implant. Water colonics are done at spas and holistic health centers using machines that very gently flow water through the intestines and then drain it out. The machines have a clear glass panel that allows you to watch the poop as it flows out. The treatment ends when the draining water is clear.

The first time you have one, the practitioner told me, you won't get all the material out. The body allows more water each time and, after three of these, you are thoroughly cleaned out. She shared an interesting factoid: "the colon by itself, weighs 5-12 lbs. but at autopsy, it weighs more like 20-25 lbs. That is because you build up all this material along the sides of the colon through your life." I asked if the typical cleaning you do before a colonoscopy brings the same result. She said to a degree it does. But it would take multiple cleanings and the materials typically used for a "clean out" before colonoscopy are very harsh on your insides and not as effective as the water colonics. You do not have to do this every time you do a transplant, only prior to the first time!

So, I highly recommend these as they are definitely easier on your body than the typical chemical colon preps and probably more thorough.

Having had this experience myself, as well as having typical bowel prep for colonoscopy, I found the water colonic to be gentle with no side effects and painless. If you have gut issues this is the way to go for bowel prep. These machines used to be traditional in all GI doctors' offices. But they take time to use and are not cost effective for today's profit-oriented medical business models. Fasting or low-fiber liquid diets before cleansing will also help.

Again, it is not necessary, and in fact, not advised to do this before subsequent transplants as you don't want to dislodge the initial transplanted microbes.

Should you proceed if you are having a "flare"?

If you have IBD take whatever medication you know will control the inflammation before FMT. **Do not do FMT in a flare unless you have no choice. Glenn Taylor, Director of Taymount says that, in his experience, trying to use FMT to control a flare is useless and advises that you use medication to calm the flare first or wait until it has subsided before proceeding with FMT.** If you have IBD, you may find the Briggs Protocol, (see Appendix D) to be helpful in calming flares prior to FMT.

Are you going to use an enema bag or enema bottle or syringe?

You can use either an old- fashioned rubber enema bag with tubing, hung on a towel rack or hook on the wall, to get gravity to work in your favor, or a disposable enema bottle (like Fleet's for example) or a plastic rectal syringe with some clear plastic catheter tubing attached. (See illustrations in Appendices.) The clinic at Taymount and the clinic in the Bahamas Medical Center use plastic rectal syringes and clear plastic catheter tubing. The tubing can be inserted a few inches more (four to six inches) than an enema bottle nozzle. It also gives you an extra push from gravity.

Personally, I use a disposable enema bottle. I found the enema bag with tubing methods difficult (for a clumsy person like myself) and prone to accidents. In using the disposable enema bottle (Fleet's, cleaned out) I did have a positive reaction so I know it can work. Look online and in medical supply stores.

People who have administered FMT to their own very young children recommend the syringe and tubing method.

Also, you are using a very small amount of implant and if you lose it, (as I did, fumbling with tubing, it won't work.) The most important thing will be to be able to perform this comfortably and stay lying down for at least thirty minutes post insertion, preferably with legs up, to allow gravity to do its work.

My strong advice is to experiment with both methods (using just distilled water) a week or so before you actually try it with a transplant. Pretend you are handling real fecal material and walk through the whole procedure a few times so you can perform it easily, without loss of material. This will determine which of the supplies you will need.

Decide if you are going to use distilled water or saline to mix with your implant.

Opinions differ which is better so you may have to experiment. Some have reported that saline has a laxative effect. Others have reported that saline is easier to hold in. The professional clinics use saline. (Saline eyewash can be used but only if it does not have any other ingredients, ie: no preservatives.)

Decide where you will do your FMT.

You can try an empty bathtub or lying on a towel on the bathroom floor. Avoid doing it on a bed or sofa or in a carpeted area in case you have a spill. I personally put a rug down on the bathroom floor covered with a plastic sheet in case of spills.

CHAPTER THIRTEEN

Timeline and Supplies

Timeline

Some preparation for your first FMT needs to start weeks ahead of time. Here is a rough timeline. Make sure you have read the decisions in section above first.

Timeline	
Two weeks before FMT	Purchase supplies.
Two weeks	Try a dry run (or several) with your enema bottle, bag or a syringe and tubing (using just saline water) and decide on the method that works best for you. You want your first procedure to go smoothly.
Two weeks	Low fiber diet (not critical) if your health issue includes bacteria that feed on starch or fiber. If you have a history of yeast infections, take sugar and high-calorie carbs out of your diet now *and* after your FMT.

Two weeks	Stop all antibiotics (critical.) If at all possible, stop earlier.
One week	If using an enema bag, hang a heavy duty adhesive hook on the wall at a height that will allow for the tube to reach your body without too much slack. Too high and the tube will not reach. Too low and you won't get enough flow from gravity.
One week	Leave plastic tubs with donor and set up transport arrangements including icepacks.
Three days	If you intend to freeze stool, plan how you will obtain and safely handle dry ice and where you will store the frozen stool. Leave plastic food containers or Ziploc bags with your donor for collection of sample.
Three days	Stop using hemorrhoid creams or suppositories before FMT as it can line the intestines and make it difficult for bacteria to adhere.
Three days	For your first FMT treatment only-have two water colonics treatments or other clean out as you would for a colonoscopy test. (Do not do this before future transplants as it will dislodge the transplanted material.)
Day of treatment	Get dry ice in place, obtain donation, if not previously frozen
Two hours	If using frozen stool, set it out at room temperature to defrost slowly.
Two hours	Get out supplies and set up your workspace.
Two hours	Try to have a bowel movement and empty your bladder. Do not eat anything that might initiate a bowel movement.

Supplies

Some people use blenders to mix stool- but I believe this puts too much air in contact with stool which promotes deterioration of bacteria.

Equipment you need, ITS NOT AS COMPLEX AS IT LOOKS!!

- **Latex free, non-powdered gloves** if you like. I do not use them as I find them too cumbersome.
- Fleet Brand (or other) **disposable enema bottles** (thoroughly rinsed free of saline) or
- Reusable Enema Bags or plastic cylinder rectal syringes and plastic tubing (available at medical supply stores.)
- **Plastic drape** to lay on floor or bed you will recline on. You can buy thin plastic tablecloths at dollar stores.
- **Measuring cup**, preferably glass, with a lip for pouring.
- **A&D ointment** or other lubricant
- Adhesive **hooks** to hang enema bag on if needed
- Fine **strainer,** preferably one that will fit on top of the measuring cup. (Also found these at the dollar store, used as kitchen drain strainers.)
- Metal **spoon** to push stool through strainer.
- **Glycerin** (from the pharmacy, to add to stool if freezing transplants.)
- **Dry ice** (necessary only if you are going to quickly freeze extra transplants.)
- Styrofoam **cooler** for dry ice if used.
- **Plastic containers with lids,** about four inches by four inches, to collect stool donation and transport.
- **Plastic wrap** to cover stool and protect from air.
- **Plastic Ziploc bags**, sandwich size.
- Saline solution or **distilled water.** (Should have no preservatives added. You can use saline eye wash- if it is *only* water and saline.)

- Small **scissors** to cut open saline packaging.
- **Timer,** watch or cell phone.
- **Trash can** with plastic liner.
- **Bimuno powder** or other prebiotic powder to add to the implant just before transplant. At the clinics you will get a tiny dose of this powder mixed in with the implant just prior to the procedure. This is to "feed" the bacteria and encourage it to grow. You can also eat a small amount before the procedure for the same purpose. One small packet is all you will need. This is optional. Available at: https://www.bimuno.com/probiotics-prebiotics. Side effect of minor gas and bloating.
- **Hydrogen peroxide** for cleanup. (It is always possible to transmit some type of illness, but the exposure to FMT is very similar to the everyday risks involved in changing diapers.) Clean up materials: hot water, soap, white vinegar or hydrogen peroxide. (Note: If you use hydrogen peroxide to clean your utensils and materials, you leave it wet on the utensils for ten minutes or more and then dry. You cannot use them for another 48 hours as the residue from the peroxide will kill good bacteria.) You can also simply pour boiling water over them after washing with soap and water.
- **Print out the instructions**, so you have them with you, especially for first time use.

Set Up For FMT

It is very important to have everything you will need to use, set up and in place ahead of time. That way, when your transplant is available, you can immediately use it.

Some people want a bed to lie on afterward, but I did the whole procedure, including the resting phase, in my bathroom on the floor. I laid an old rug down and put the plastic over the rug. I put a pillow (inside a plastic garbage bag) at one end and a folded towel (for my back or rear end) at the other end. It is a good idea to have a practice run with all of this before you try it with a transplant in hand. I put my cell phone close at hand to use as a timer and a box of Kleenex on the floor. I lined the trash can with a plastic bag so that all disposables could be bagged and discarded without getting the trash can dirty. I wore older clothes (that I don't mind getting messed up) on my upper body so I will be warm enough.

It is best to choose a time when you are less inflamed or having less diarrhea. But if you are working on your donor's schedule you may not be able to pick the day or time.

If you will be using frozen material, two hours before your procedure, defrost it at room temperature. This should take about two hours. You can help this by placing the bag of material in a cup of tepid (never hot!) water.

If you can have a bowel movement before you start the treatment, that would be helpful. It is also a good idea not to eat or drink a big meal that may induce a bowel movement later or drink anything that will make you have to urinate frequently.

Taymount recommends a prebiotic diet or using small amounts (1/4 teaspoon) of a prebiotic powder like Bimuno (https://www.bimuno.com/) the day of the transplant to feed the new bacteria and initiate its growth. You can also add some of this (about a third of a small sachet) to your transplant material just before implanting it.

For your first time with FMT it may be best to use fresh, unfrozen stool. Many people report they get a better result from fresh stool. You will not know how well FMT can work for you without having this comparison. However, the professional clinics only use frozen. If you are using fresh transplant, it must be used or frozen within 2-3 hours of being expelled. During those hours, it should be kept cold, not hot.

CHAPTER FOURTEEN

Step by Step FMT Instructions

You have your donor. He or she has been tested and found to be clear of pathogens as well as having a healthy microbial diversity. You and your donor have discussed the logistics and made arrangements for dropping off the stool. You have had your clean out. You have talked with your doctor, done your pre-FMT arrangements for diet/antimicrobials etc. You have tried a trial run or two to perfect your technique. Now that you have all the research and pre-FMT work done...**you are ready to do your first FMT.**

1. Instructions for the donor: If possible, **collect stool directly into a plastic container**. No urine should be mixed in. No water, no soap. Do not use stool if it has fallen into the toilet water. Place a piece of plastic wrap over the stool to protect it from the air, then put lid on the container. **Place it in a Styrofoam cooler** (or other container) with ice packs around it. Donee must use or freeze within two-three hours of collection. If for any reason, you cannot meet that deadline, put

the stool in the refrigerator until you can use it. After three hours it may have lost much of its benefit.

2. If using frozen stool, take it out to **defrost two hours ahead of time. Do not defrost by heating- this will kill bacteria.**

3. If you are using fresh stool and would like to freeze some of the stool, separate that out and **spoon into a plastic zip-lock bag, add a few drops of glycerin, squeeze the bag to mix glycerin in with stool and seal.** Place in dry ice to quickly freeze. Once frozen, you can put in a regular refrigerator freezer. (Never put dry ice in your freezer as it will damage it.)

4. Take a small portion of fresh stool—maybe a half of a cup. **Push stool through the fine strainer into the measuring cup,** using a spoon to help compress it. Keep adding stool and mashing it through the strainer.

5. You will have to **add small amounts of saline water** or distilled water to move it through the mesh sieve. (The water should not be cold or hot, just tepid.) Use as little water as possible at this point. Just enough to get the stool through the strainer. You should wind up with approximately three and a half ounces or no more than 100 milliliters of fine liquid. Less is OK. The amount of transplant you wind up with is not critical, more is not necessarily better as too much liquid will only act as an enema and induce a bowel movement. Use tissue to clean out strainer and spoon of stool and debris that won't easily go through. Discard tissue in toilet.

6. Make sure that your liquid material is **fine enough to pass through the enema bottle nozzle freely**. If too thick, add very small amounts of distilled water or saline solution and mix with spoon.

7. **Pour the material into the enema bottle, bag or rectal syringe**. If using an enema bag with tubing, hang it on a hook and make sure the clamp is squeezed shut (or the material will

flow right out of it!) Make sure all the air is out of the tube before insertion. You do not want to pump yourself up with air.

8. **Put the enema bottle or enema bag, bottle, syringe and tubing where you can reach it when lying down.**

9. **Insert a dab of A&D ointment or other lubricant into your anus.** Lay down on your left side on the floor (or bed).) Elevate your butt, either with a pillow (I put my pillow inside a plastic garbage bag first to keep it clean) or folded towel. Make gravity your friend.

10. Once you are set and comfortable, **insert the bottle nozzle or tubing into your anus.** If using tubing make sure it stays on the syringe tip.

11. **Slowly squeeze the enema bottle or syringe**. (Or release the clamp on the tubing if using an enema bag.) If nothing comes out of the enema bottle, you may want to remove the backflow valve from the enema bottle and try again. (This is a small round piece of plastic that stops liquid from going back into the bottle.) If it is still not coming out move your position slightly and try again. You should feel a cool sensation as the transplant comes into you. Make sure that the bottle will be higher than your butt. Never force it. Slight discomfort may be normal but it should not be painful. Stop if it is painful.

12. **Relax, take a deep breath and continue until the bottle or bag is empty.** This should be done gradually. You can take breaks.

13. If you feel like you are going to expel it, **stop and try to hold in what you have**. You can wait a bit and try again. Put a tissue against your rectum to protect against leaks.

14. Then, **lay on your left side with butt elevated for at least ten minutes** or more. Massage your abdomen to push the FMT gently up your colon. Then lie on your back for another ten minutes or longer. Lay on your stomach for ten minutes.

Then on your right side for ten more. Then on your stomach for ten more. The longer you can rest in these positions the more chance the bacteria has to make its way through the colon and attach to the colon walls. Try to stay down at least forty minutes.

15. Congratulations, you have done it!

16. You may be able to get up and retain the transplant for four hours or more, or you may lose it almost immediately. To avoid losing it, **try not to sit on the toilet or do anything that would initiate a bowel movement**, like drinking hot coffee or eating a heavy meal. If you do lose it don't worry, as it takes very little bacteria a short time to populate your colon.

17. If you are using a re-useable enema bag, there are several ways to clean it. You can use very hot water and soap or wash it out then rinse with hydrogen peroxide. If you use the peroxide, let it dry without rinsing. If you use peroxide and let it dry in the enema bag, you will not be able to use the enema bag for 48 hours so you do not kill the bacteria in the next implant. One of the many reasons I prefer the disposable enema bottle or the plastic syringe.

CHAPTER FIFTEEN

After Your First FMT

Common reactions

Initial reactions may include cramping, gas, diarrhea as your body adjusts to the new bacteria. In some cases, the bad bacteria die-off causes symptoms that may make you feel worse temporarily. In patients with colitis and Crohn's, pain in the abdomen and fatigue can result after FMT as the strains of bacteria battle it out. Continue with the FMT infusions.

Care and feeding after your first FMT

- Do not undertake any special diets/antimicrobials and especially no antibiotics after the first FMT, unless you are instructed to do so by your physician.
- Only take a fiber supplement if you cannot get enough fiber through your diet. If you have IBD you will need to go easy

on the fiber until your gut wall can cope, and then introduce it only slowly.

- A high fiber diet will help grow new microbiota in some people, but don't overdo it. Not all fibers agree with all people. Continue with your regular diet in the first days of fecal transplants, then slowly add in fiber foods to see how you react. Experiment until you find the right ones. Some of the top prebiotic fiber foods include: chicory root, Jerusalem Artichoke, dandelion greens, garlic, leeks, onion, asparagus (raw is best.)

- Do not use starchy fiber if your condition is autism, myalgic encephalopathy or chronic fatigue syndrome. Research is showing that these conditions produce too many fatty acids (and possibly the wrong kind) from their microbiome. You do not want to feed your new FMT microbiome starch if you have those conditions as it may encourage the *wrong* bacteria to grow.

- If you have food intolerances don't try anything that isn't a known safe food (or supplement), for at least 3 months after FMT and then only introduce slowly.

- If you experience die-off or side effects, try a liver tonic to support your liver which may be under pressure from the readjustment occurring in your gut.

- If you suffer from intestinal permeability (leaky gut) try one of the repair formulas available. It might take a few to find one that has the right mix of ingredients for you. Restore is an excellent leaky-gut remedy. Perm-a-Vit and Intestinew have a good mix of gut healing ingredients. Customized formulas are also available from some naturopathic practitioners.

- Get your zinc levels tested and make sure they are on the high side of normal. Zinc is essential for healing. Zinc Lozenges are better than tablets as they bypass the digestive system.

- If you have IBD, read the Briggs Protocol which contains a step by step gut repair strategy.

- If FMT doesn't work for you, try a different donor or investigate factors that might be disrupting growth of the new flora.
- You may want to record the dates you do transplants and what your reaction is that day and the next day. Look at your stool for changes and note them. Changes may not be noticeable for three months or more. Keeping a diary of symptoms is very useful.

How many times should you do fecal transplants?

Research has indicated the following:

- Clostridium Difficile (C.diff) tend to get positive results within 1-3 transplants.
- IBS & SIBO tend to get positive results within 3-10 transplants
- IBD tend to get positive results if they use it daily for a few weeks or a month, then taper off to once a week and then once a month. There are several protocols being used by doctors/ clinics. Take a look at Taymount and Newbery Clinics for suggestions.
- For conditions like ulcerative colitis, clinical trials of eight weeks of FMT daily or more have had success. (FMT five times a week for eight or more weeks.) In these trials, remission lasted through a five year follow up. (See the sections in this book on digestive and autoimmune diseases and clinical trials using FMT.)
- People with other health issues will need to experiment. This is a new therapy and we don't have all the answers. One option is to look up your condition on Google Scholar and include the term fecal transplant to see most current research on FMT and your health condition.

CHAPTER SIXTEEN

The Future

The Future

Right now, companies like Open Biome have made material needed for FMT transplants available to any physician in the United States. Donor testing can be obtained by anyone who wants it and is willing to pay for it.

Studies show FMT is a safe and simple procedure with few side effects. An abundance of clinical trials and studies in this country and abroad prove that not only is FMT the preferred cure for C. diff. infections but it can bring about remission in diseases like colitis when performed over an extended period of time. Numerous physician reports also indicate FMT may be important in correcting the causal factors in many autoimmune illnesses. The opportunities are wide open for FMT to become mainstream with a small assist from the FDA.

Beyond acceptance of FMT as a therapy, the future of gut biology is full of possibilities. In particular, immunotherapy for cancers has been shown to have a stronger response in patients with healthy and diverse microbiomes. Scientists are beginning to match the lack of or abundance of specific bacteria strains to specific diseases. This matching will allow fine tuning of designer probiotics for various conditions. Clinics, many of them trained by the staff at Taymount Clinic in the U.K., are opening up across Europe. The possibilities are exciting.

Clearly, the newfound relevance of the bacteria that lives inside us and runs our brains and immune systems, should lead us to focus hard on ways to make this valuable part of the body healthier and stronger. The care and feeding of our microbiome as well as procedures such as fecal microbiota transplant may be the most important topics for us to utilize in our battles to regain health and keep it.

Now we have a better understanding of the critical value of these tiny life forms within us., a realization too, that the *external* environment is impacting heavily on our *internal* environment and thus, our health. Keeping the gut healthy in the first place, after all, may prevent many of the diseases that currently plague us.

What You Can Do to Help

Call the FDA and ask for a public hearing on the subject of fecal transplant availability and access to FMT through your local gastrointestinal doctor. Talk to your GI doc about FMT, ask him if he would be willing to write to the FDA or attend a hearing if they have one. Share whatever information has been helpful to you to others, especially those with diseases like Chron's and colitis.

You can donate to the Fecal Transplant Foundation: thefecal-transplantfoundation.org/

You can donate to the Power of Poop website which provides updated current information on FMT here are around the world. Thepowerofpoop.com

THE CATHERINE DUFF STORY

Catherine Duff is part of the history of fecal transplant and hopefully, part of the future. FMT saved her life when she was suffering from a severe, long term C.diff infection her doctors were not able to cure. There is also her plea to the FDA to allow use of FMT for C.diff and possibly other health conditions. I would second that plea. The more that FMT is used for conditions we know it cures (like C.diff) and the more that doctors are allowed to use it for conditions where research has shown that it can bring about long term cure without harmful side effects, (like colitis), the more we will learn about this valuable therapy. With the rate of autoimmune disease rising rapidly, this understanding is urgently needed. Here is her story as published on the website of the Fecal Transplant Foundation (www.fecaltransplant foundation.org)

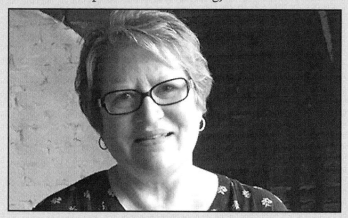

Catherine Duff
(Photo: permission of Catherine Duff) http://fecaltransplant.org/)

IN HER OWN WORDS

"Many of you will be familiar with my story; the months, years really, spent lying in bed without the energy to do anything. Feeling my life slip away and being helpless to alter the outcome, and of beginning to reach the surreal point where I realized I wasn't sure I cared anymore; I was just too tired of being sick and living, or not living, this way.

After my successful Fecal Microbiota Transplant (FMT) I started The Fecal Transplant Foundation as a way to reach out to other patients, physicians, clinicians, scientists, researchers, investigators, and regulatory agencies about this life saving treatment.

Shortly afterward, I attended the FDA/CBER FMT Public Workshop in Bethesda, MD, on May 2nd and 3rd, 2013. After realizing I was the only patient, and the only actual member of the "public" in attendance among the approximately one hundred and fifty (150) participants, I felt compelled to speak out about the impact this treatment had on my life and could have on the millions of people not being represented there. Following my talk, many of the physicians in the audience reached out to me, and I, in turn, reached out to others, and what resulted, in a remarkably short period of time, was the assemblage of a prestigious group of leaders in the field of FMT, as well as a few others who have volunteered or been asked to help, because they all want to move the science of this treatment forward, and to make it more accessible for patients, and providers.

Below is the transcript of my remarks as they were intended to be made at the FDA/CBER FMT Public Workshop in May 2013. In reality, I was crying and very emotional and unable to read the complete version, but I think I hit the high points. The entire

800 pages of the transcript of the two day workshop is available at: http://thefecaltransplantfoundation.org/founders-message/.

"Hi. My name is Catherine Duff, and no, I'm not from around here. I seem to be the only actual member of the public present at this Public Workshop, and, at the risk of annoying those of you who are hoping to avoid a long commute, I think at least one member of the public should be heard here, and I have a brief statement.

To start, I would like to clarify that I have no affiliations with anyone or anything related to this, that I was not invited here by anyone, and none of my expenses have been paid by anyone other than myself.

I am one of the people who have called or emailed too many doctors to count. I have had 8 episodes of increasingly severe and prolonged C. diff. since 2005. It is now antibiotic resistant. I began considering FMT after learning of it not from any of my team of excellent physicians, but from one of my daughters, a corporate tax attorney in DC, who loves to do research for fun.

I took our googled recipe, protocol and stack of research papers to each of my physicians. Only two had even heard of FMT, and none had performed it. These physicians, to a person, were denied permission to perform FMT by their practice partners or affiliated hospitals, respectively, citing liability concerns, without even knowing what an IND was, that it was required, or that a CPT code had been assigned.

My husband and I performed FMT by enema, at home, in March, 2012, after one of my physicians agreed to write the order for my husband's stool test.

Within 24 hours, all symptoms disappeared, and two weeks later no C. diff. or toxins were detected. I remained free of C. diff. until last summer. By last fall, one of my physicians had convinced his partners to allow him to perform FMT, again without knowing what an IND was or that one was needed, or that a CPT code had been assigned. Again, within 24 hours, all symptoms were gone, and I have remained asymptomatic and toxin free since. The physician's practice has since been purchased by a healthcare system, and he is no longer allowed to perform FMTs.

People are desperate for this treatment. As doctors, clinicians, researchers, and administrators, you all know the stories of C. diff. patients, but you have not lived our lives nor felt our dwindling hope and growing sense of despair and helplessness. I now wonder each and every day if I will be able to have another FMT if needed, what I will do if FMT ceases to work, and knowing what will happen to me if I encounter a different superbug."[102]

Suggestions from the Fecal Transplant Foundation

Contact your U.S. Senators & U.S. Representatives and tell them you want increased funding for FMT Research.

Contact the Funding Division of NIH, (National Institutes of Health), which is responsible for granting all U.S. government medical research dollars and let them know you support increased funding for FMT.

Contact the (NIH) National Center for Advancing Translational Sciences (NCATS). The mission of the NCATS is to catalyze the generation of innovative methods and technologies that will enhance the development, testing, and implementation of diagnostics and therapeutics across a wide range of human diseases and conditions. Please contact them and let them know you support increased funding for FMT.

Illustrations

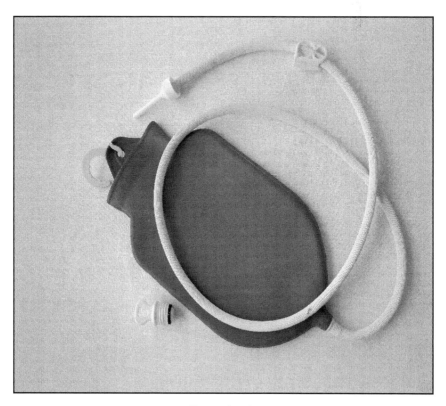

Enema bottle
Photo: D.York

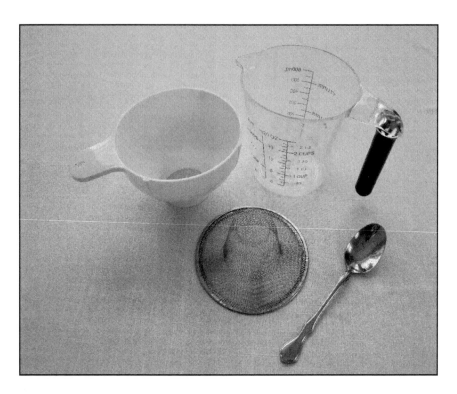

Measuring cup, funnel, mesh strainer, spoon for mixing and refining stool.
Photo: D. York

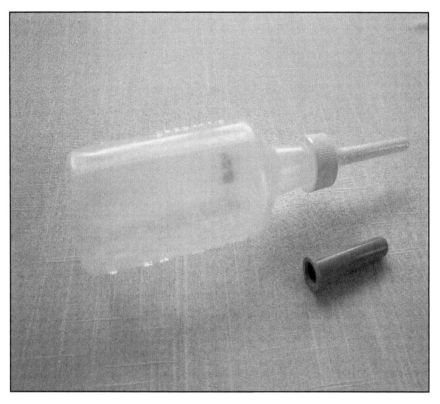

Disposable Enema Bottle
Photo: D. York

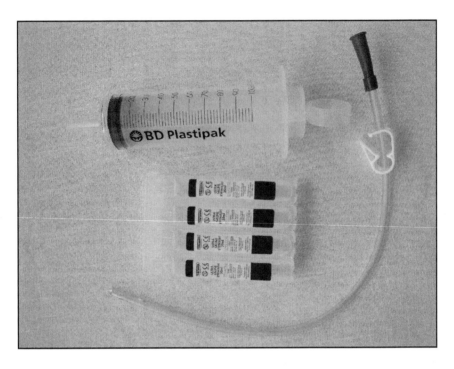

Syringe, tubing, clamp and saline packets
Photo D. York

The Bristol Stool Chart

Type 1		Separate hard lumps, like nuts (hard to pass)
Type 2		Sausage-shaped but lumpy
Type 3		Like a sausage but with cracks on the surface
Type 4		Like a sausage or snake, smooth and soft
Type 5		Soft blobs with clear-cut edges
Type 6		Fluffy pieces with ragged edges, a mushy stool
Type 7		Watery, no solid pieces. **Entirely Liquid**

Reprinted with permission of the Rome Foundation
(theromefoundation.org)

Donor Questionnaire

(By permission from the Power of Poop website, thepowerofpoop.com)

Donor Screening Questionnaire for Fecal Microbiota Transplant Donors.

1. Do you have any chronic illnesses?

2. Do you have any autoimmune conditions (e.g.. Grave's disease, IBD, lupus, rheumatoid arthritis, other)?

3. Do you have irritable bowel syndrome or suffer from diarrhea or constipation often?

4. Do you take medication on a daily basis?
   a. If yes, which medications and for what reason?

5. Have you taken antibiotics in the last 6 months?
   a. If yes, why?

6. Do you smoke?

7. Have you ever used drugs intravenously?

8. Have you ever had a tattoo?

9. Have you ever been rejected as a blood donor?
   a. If yes, why?

10. Have you ever received blood products or a blood transfusion?
    a. If yes, where and when?

11. Have you ever received any type of transplant (e.g. organ, tissue, cornea, hair, etc.)? a. If yes, where, when, and what type?

12. Were you born in a country outside the United States, or have you ever resided in a country outside the U.S. for more than 1 year?
    a. If yes, when and where?

13. Have you traveled outside of the U.S. in the last two years?
    a. If yes, where and when?

14. Have you ever had malaria?
    a. If yes, when?

15. Have you received vaccinations for hepatitis B?

16. While visiting another country (for work or vacation), have you ever had sexual contact with people originating from that country?
    a. If yes, when and where?

17. Do you have a new sexual partner with whom you have commenced sexual relations within the last 12 months?

18. Have you ever had anonymous sexual contacts?

19. Have you ever had sexual contact with someone who uses IV drugs?

20. Have you ever had sexual contact with someone of your own sex?

21. Have you ever had sexual contact with a bisexual or homosexual man?

22. In the last 12 months, have you had receptive anal sex with a new partner?

23. Have you ever had sexual contact with someone who received money from you for this contact?

24. Have you ever worked as a prostitute?

25. Have you ever had sexual contact with someone who turned out to be infected with HIV, HTLV, hepatitis, or syphilis?
    a. If yes, which ones?

26. Have you ever had a sexually transmittable disease (e.g. HIV, syphilis, hepatitis B, hepatitis C, gonorrhea, chlamydia, genital herpes, trichomonas, bacterial vaginosis, HPV, other)?

27. Have you ever been treated for an intestinal infection (e.g. C. difficile, Salmonella, Shigella, Campylobacter, Yersinia, E. coli, rotavirus, norovirus, intestinal parasites, other)?
    a. If yes, which ones and when?

28. Do you have hemorrhoids?

29. Have you ever had blood in your stools? a. If yes, were any extra tests performed? What were the results?

30. Have you had a fever in the past two weeks?

31. What is your profession?

Note: questionnaire adapted and modified from Michael Docktor, personal communication and van Nood E, Vrieze A, Nieuwdorp M, et al. Duodenal infusion of donor feces for recurrent Clostridium difficile. N Engl J Med 2013;368:407-15.

List of Physicians in USA who are FMT Providers:

(As stated previously, these physicians can treat C.diff. cases only or give assistance in testing.)

Alabama

Joseph Brasco MD, Huntsville, AL

Arizona

Mayo Clinic in Phoenix AZ

Andrew Weinberg MD, Gilbert AZ

California

Purety Family Medical Clinic, Santa Barbara, CA

Shelley Gordon MD, California Pacific Medical CA

Alister George MD, Thousand Oaks, CA

Neil Stollman MD, Oakland, CA (C. diff only. Doen't help with DIY)

Allen Kamrava MD, Beverly Hills, CA

Los Angeles Colon and Rectal Surgical Associates CA

KT Park MD, Palo Alto, CA (pediatrics)

Colorado

Steve Freeman, MD, University of Colorado

Florida

Jose Vasquez, MD, Brandon, FL

Lawrence Fielder MD, Boca Raton, FL

Sovi Joseph, Port Charlotte, FL

Katherine A. Kosche, MD, Pembroke Pines, FL

RDS Infusions, Tampa FL (David Shepard MD—will consult for other conditions)

Georgia

Tanvi Dhere, MD, Johns Ck, GA

Jeffrey D. Lewis, MD, GA — (pediatrics)

Satish M Rao, M.D. Augusta, GA

Douglas Wolf St. Joseph, Atlanta GA

Illinois

Eugene F Yen MD , Evanston, IL

David Rubin, MD, Chicago IL

Prabhakar Swaroop, M.D Chicago IL

Louisiana

Arnab Ray MD, New Orleans, LA

Massachusetts

Brian Gill MD, Plymouth, MA .

Maryland

Maria Oliva-Hemker, M.D. John Hopkins Children's Hospital Baltimore, MD

Maria Oliva-Hemka MD, Baltimore MD (Paediatrician)

Sudhir K. Dutta MD, Baltimore MD

Michael J. Docktor, Boston MD (IBD Pediatrician)

Minnesota

Tim Rubin MD, Minnesota

Mayo Clinic Minnesota

Alexander Khoruts MD, Minneapolis MN

Darrell Pardi, MD / Sahil Khanna, MMS Mayo Clinic,
Rochester, MN

Missouri

Jack Bragg and Dr. Ghassan Hammoud, University of Missouri
Health Center, Columbia, MO

Montana

William M. Chamberlin, MD, Billings MT

North Carolina

Martin H Poleski, MD, CM Durham, NC

Robert T Elliot MD, Burlington, NC

Barry Schneider MD, Charlotte, NC

New Hampshire

Susan Edwards DHMC, Lebanon, NH (pediatrics)

New Jersey

Robert W. Schuman MD, West Orange, NJ

Kevin S. Skole, MD, Plainsboro, NJ

New Mexico

Daniel Hamptom, MD, Las Cruces, NM

Daniel Hampton MD, Las Cruces, NM, USA

Nevada

Gastroenterology Consultants, Reno, NV

New York

Ellen Scherl, MD, NY NY .
Caterina Oneto, MD, NYU School of Medicine
Lawrence Brandt, New York, NY
Lee Ann Chen MD, NY, NY
Caterina Oneto, MD, NY, NY
Jonathan Goldstein MD, Rochester, NY
Lisa B Malter, NY NY

Ohio

Ohio Hospitals

Oklahoma

Mark Mellow MD, Oklahoma City OK

Oregon

Bright Medicine Clinic, Portland, OR (Mark Davis ND—will consult on other issues)
Microbiomes LLC, Portland, OR (Carmen Campbell ND & Mark Davis ND)
Paul F Schleinitz MD, Oregon

Pennsylvania

Alka Goyal, MD, Pittsburgh, PA (pediatrician)
Jackson Seigelbaum, MD, Gastroenterology Harrisburg, PA
Drexel Medicine, Philadelphia, PA & other locations

Rhode Island

Colleen Kelly MD. Rhode Island

South Carolina

Gordon France, Spartanburg Regional, SC
Joseph Baber DO FACP, Greenville, SC

Tennessee

Michael Vaezi, MD, Nashville, TN

Mahdi M. Budayr, MD, Maryville, TN

Dr. Sara Horst and Dr. Dawn Beaulieu through Vanderbilt IBD Clinic, Nashville, TN

Maribeth Nicholson, MD Nashville, TN (pediatrics)

Texas

F. Lyone Hochman, MD, Houston, TX

Melvin K Lau MD and Dr Vu Nhu Nguyen MD, Round Rock, TX

Utah

John F. Pohl MD, Salt Lake City, UT (Pediatrician)

Virginia

David A Johnson MD, Norfolk, VA

Washington

David L Suskind MD, Seattle, WA (pediatrics)

Christina M Surawicz, MD Seattle, WA (pediatrics)

Roy Ozanne MD, Langley, WA

US PHYSICIANS –
BOARD OF ADVISORS TO THE FECAL TRANSPLANT FOUNDATION

Dr. Mark Davis, N.D., Naturopathic Physician

The Bright Medicine Clinic

Portland OR

Dr. Colleen Kelly, MD, Gastroenterologist

Clinical Assistant Professor of Medicine

Brown University, Alpert Medical School

Division of Gastroenterology—Liver Research Center

Women's Medicine Collaborative

Providence RI

Dr. Alexander Khoruts, MD, Gastroenterologist, Immunologist
Associate Professor of Medicine, University of Minnesota
Division of Gastroenterology Center for Immunology, Microbiology
Immunology and Cancer Biology Graduate Program
Minneapolis MN

Dr. Stacy Kahn, M.D, Pediatric Gastroenterologist
Assistant Professor of Pediatrics & Medicine, Director, Transitional
IBD Clinic, Section of Pediatric Gastroenterology, Hepatology, &
Nutrition,
The University of Chicago, Chicago IL

International List of Providers

ARGENTINA

Dr. Silvio Najt
Newbery Medicine
Jorge Newbery 3571, Floor 2, Apt. 2 (C1427EGN)
Buenos Aires, Argentina
http://newberymedicine.com
info@newberymedicine.com
(They can perform four weeks of treatment and accept other
disorders than C.diff., Very reasonable cost)

AUSTRALIA

Dr. Thomas Borody, M.D.
The Center for Digestive Diseases
Level 1, 229 Great North Road
Five Dock NSW, 2046 Australia
Phone: 61-2-9713-4011, Fax: 61-2-9712-1675
http://www.cdd.com.au
(Note: They will consider colitis, Crohn's and other diseases. Dr.
Borody is one of the pioneers in use of fecal transplant for C. diff.
and has conducted numerous trials with FMT for other conditions.)

Dr. Paul Froomes
Melbourne, Victoria, Australia
Phone: 61-29-331-3122
drpaulfroomes.com.au

The Centre for Digestive Diseases, Sydney, NSW
Dr Sanjay Nandurkar, Box Hill, VIC
Moonee Valley Specialist Centre, Moonee Ponds, VIC
Melbourne FMT, Moonee Ponds, VIC

BAHAMAS

Sakina Sands
International Patient Program Director
Bahamas Medical Center, Nassau, Bahamas
Phone: 866-277-5054
Email: ssands@bahamasmedicalcenter.com

CANADA (C.diff. only)

Dr. Susy Hota
University Health Network
University of Toronto
Toronto, Ontario
susy.hota@uhn.ca or maryjane.salpeter@uhn.ca

Dr. Christine Lee, M.D.
Medical Director, Infection Prevention & Control, St. Joseph's
Healthcare, Hamilton
Director, Microbiology Services, Hamilton Health Sciences and St.
Joseph's Healthcare in Hamilton
Professor, Department of Pathology and Molecular Medicine
McMaster University
50 Charlton Avenue E.
Hamilton, Ontario L8N 4A6
Phone: 905-521-6143

http://fhs.mcmaster.ca/pathology/contact_us/faculty/faculty_bios/
lee_c.html

Dr. Michael Silverman
Lakeridge Health
1 Hospital Court
Oshowa, Ontario, Canada
Phone: 905-721-4717

DENMARK

Bakterieklinikken
Bydammen 1G, 1.tv.
2750 Ballerup
info@bakterieklinikken.dk
40 74 90 77

FINLAND

Dr. Eero Mattila, M.D.
Faculty of Medicine
Helsinki University Central Hospital
Tukholmankatu 8B, 5th & 6th Floors
Helsinki, Finland
Phone: 358-9-1911

GERMANY

Medical Clinic Milz-Bieber
Unterthal 32,
Bad Grönebach, 87730
Phone: 011 49 8334 986626
Email: office1@milz-bieber.de (email sent 9/13/17)
http://www.whatclinic.com/holistic-health/germany/
bad-gronebach/medical-clinic-villa-thal

GUATEMALA

Dr. Jorge Chang Mayorga
Boulevard Vista Hermosa 25-29 Zona 15
Edificio Multimedica, Of. 806
Ciudad de Guatemala, Guatemala, C.D.
PBX: (502) 2386-7522 FAX: (502) 2386-7510
jchm1958@yahoo.com
www.gastro.com.gt
Doing FMT for C. diff. and colitis

SLOVAKIA

Institute of Predictive Personalized Medicine
Hanácka 1492/9,
821 04 Bratislava,
Slovakia
Telephone: +421 911 212 838
Email: office@ippm.sk
(Note: They do work with other disorders- they say fees are similar
to Taymount, their staff was trained by Taymount. They order
their transplants from Taymount. They usually offer a ten-day
treatment plan.

UKRAINE

Andrey E. Dorofeyev M.D., Ph.D., Dr. Med. Sci. Professor
Bogomolets National Medical University
01601, T. Shevchenko Boulevard
17 Kyiv, Ukraine
Tel: (044) 235-91-73
dorofeyev@med.finfort.co

UNITED KINGDOM

Dove Clinic in Twyford, UK
The Old Brewery
High Street
Twyford
Hampshire
SO21 1RG
Tel: 01962 718000
Fax: 01962 717060

Dove Clinic, London, UK
London Clinic
10 Harley Street
London
W1G 9PF
PH: 01962718000
secretaries@doveclinic.com

Dr. Simon Goldenberg
Directorate of Infection, Guy's & St Thomas' NHS
Foundation Trust
5th Floor North Wing
St Thomas' Hospital
Westminster Bridge Road
London SE1 7EH
UK
simon.goldenberg@gstt.nhs.uk
+44 (0)20 7188 8515

Dr. Benjamin Mullish
Academic Clinical Fellow, Gastroenterology and Hepatology
Imperial College London
10th Floor of the QEQM, Liver and Anti-Viral Centre
St Mary's Hospital
South Wharf Road
London W2 1NY
UK
Tel: +44 (0)203 312 6454
Fax: +44 (0)207 724 9369

The Taymount Clinic
16a High Street
Hitchin, Hertfordshire SG5 1AT
United Kingdom
Phone: 44-0-1462-712-500
http://www.taymount.com

The Briggs Protocol

(Reprinted with permission from Power Of Poop website)

The Briggs Protocol is a three-step process involving inducing remission, healing the gut wall and maintaining the gut wall. The following is the Briggs plan reproduced from the Power of Poop website. For additional information see: http://thepowerofpoop. com/wp-content/uploads/2015/07/IBD-Briggs-July-21-2015-1-1.pdf

Michael Briggs holds a PHD in Physics, works as a university lecturer and has recovered from 12 years of Ulcerative Colitis using this protocol. He is not a medical doctor.

When he became a father, Michael decided not to accept the mainstream medical view that he would face a lifetime of stronger and riskier immunosuppressant drugs, with all likelihood that he would eventually have his colon removed. So he did what a PHD scientist does best, he researched everything there was to know about the pathology of UC. He reviewed over 200 research papers, formulated a treatment plan and when it worked extremely well for him, decided to circulate it to other sufferers so that they, like him, would "never have to crap blood again". His gastroenterologist has been supportive and says his "biopsies are amazing".

Phase 1—Induce Remission

Remission can usually be induced with a combination of drugs and anti-oxidants. However, some of the drugs used to treat IBD can also aggravate healing of the leaky gut and are to be avoided unless absolutely necessary (prednisone in particular).

Below are the therapies that work well for Phase 1. Experiment and see which combination works best for you. If you are sensitive to supplements, then work up to the full dose gradually. See the full protocol for links to the research.

A. Anti-TNF-α therapy:

- The anti-depressant Wellbutrin (bupropion) is a TNF (tumor necrosis factor) inhibitor. It should be taken in its immediate release form, at a dosage of three 100 mg pills a day. Slow release is not as effective. Be careful with Wellbutrin if you have liver issues. Some people experience temporary side effects like nausea, insomnia, or anxiety—these generally go away after about a week.
- Curcumin and Quercetin, however studies have not yet clearly identified what dosage is required to induce remission and this will vary from person to person.
- The anti-TNF antibodies Remicade and Humira, but with a significant drawback—they are foreign proteins and your body will eventually develop antibodies to them. Also, they seem to have more side effects than Wellbutrin.

B. Boosting methylation:

Ascertain (through 23andme or other means) if there are any genetic mutations that inhibit your methylation pathways. If so, supplement with methyl folate to ensure adequate MTHFR enzyme production, to make N-acetyl Lcysteine, glutathione, phosphatidylcholine etc.

C. Hydrogen Sulfide Inhibition:

5-ASAs, such as Lialda (mesalamine) are effective at inhibiting bacterial production of hydrogen sulfide, which can help get the redox balance back under control. They are also potent anti-inflammatory agents.

D. Prescription anti-inflammatories:

Take only if necessary. Drugs like prednisone have serious side effects and should be avoided unless absolutely necessary to induce remission.

E. Natural anti-oxidants:

Vitamin E, n-Acetyl L-cysteine, glutathione, milk thistle (the active component silymarin has been shown to help with maintaining remission of UC), riboflavin (mostly to help boost concentration of Faecalibacterium prausnitzii).

F. Phosphatidylcholine:

2 grams daily until mucus and bleeding have stopped, then 1 gram daily.

G. Amino Acids:

- L-Glutamine: 10-20 grams daily. Note that some genetic mutations can result in a person having issues with excess ammonia production or glutamate related to high intake of glutamine or protein in general.
- L-glycine: 5-grams daily

H. Diet:

Reduce the ratio of pro-inflammatory Omega 6 fatty acids to anti-inflammatory Omega 3 fatty acids. Avoid the following:

- Fiber (this will be added in Phase 2 once inflammation subsides)
- High sulfur foods, sulfite and sulfur preservatives
- Protein
- Gluten (most grains)*
- Lectins (legumes, nuts and seeds)*
- Sugar
- Processed foods containing additives
- Any foods that you have a high IgA response to. If you can't afford IgA testing, be vigilant and monitor your diet for irritants. Be that aware corn, soy and dairy are big offenders.

The toxic properties of foods marked with an asterix above can be reduced by sprouting the grains and soaking the nuts, seeds, and legumes in a process called 'activation' (while soaking, phytic acid and lectins are broken down and released). These foods can be introduced in their activated form in Phase 3. Some grains, in particular millet, sorghum, and white rice have minimal lectin activity and don't seem to need special treatment.

Note though that gluten should continue to be avoided for the rest of your life. Gluten has been shown to trigger an immediate leaky gut in everyone, whether they have celiac disease or not (it just lasts longer in people with celiac). We want to avoid that at all costs.

I. Avoid fluoridated water:

Fluoride depletes ATP from epithelial cells, reducing their energy reserves.

J. Anti-inflammatory enemas:

- 3,000 to 7,000 IUs of natural vitamin E
- 500 mg of reduced glutathione
- 1 gram of colostrum
- 500 mg of phosphatidylcholine
- 5 grams of L-glutamine
- 50 mL of water.

Anti-inflammatory enemas should be undertaken until inflammation has cleared. They are best done before bed to help with retention. Note that since inflamed tissue is ineffective at absorbing water and vitamin E has a mild laxative effect, these enemas will likely result in a loose stool in the morning—but it will still help get the inflammation under control. It can be more effective to make suppositories by mixing a reduced amount of the ingredients in melted cocoa butter and pouring into the fingers of a latex glove and refrigerating.

K. Probiotics:

- Lactobacillus Rhamnosus GG ("Culturelle")
- Lactobacillus plantarum
- Clostridium butyricum miyairi
- Digestive Advantage Daily Probiotic (to boost Faecalibacterium prausnitzii)

All have been found effective at inhibiting the inflammatory response in IBD. It is important to avoid a dramatic introduction of diverse microbiota (such as in fecal transplants) while inflamed and flaring as the gut wall may reject the new microbiota or react violently. Fecal transplants are best done after inflammation is under control, however these particular probiotics can be taken during Phase 1.

L. Reduce Stress:

- Mindfulness Meditation
- Whatever practice you know works best for you.
- No excuses. Nothing is more important than your health.

Phase 2: Heal the Gut Wall

Do not move to Phase 2 until your inflammation has stopped (no more mucus or bleeding). Below are the therapies that work well for Phase 1. Experiment and see which combination works best for you. If you are sensitive to supplements, then work up to the full dose gradually. See the full protocol for links to the research.

A. Diet:

A probiotic diet rich in fiber and resistant starch should be adopted once inflammation is under control, but not before. To be safe, start out slowly and work up to higher levels. Ultimately your diet should include significant levels of fiber and resistant starches for production of SCFAs (short chain fatty acids), in particular butyrate. This also feeds beneficial anaerobic bacteria that help down-regulate the immune response in the gut. Consume vegetables for fiber and beans and rice for resistant starches (soak the beans for several hours and cook thoroughly to break down lectins and phytic acid).

In addition to introducing high fiber foods, you can also supplement with 15-20 grams of fiber per day, such as inulin, fructo-oligosaccharides, oligofructose, plus 1-2 grams of chitosan oligosaccharide. Follow the other dietary restrictions in Phase 1, but increasing protein a little, which is required for cell repair. In Phase 3 you will introduce more protein, but for now it should be on the lower side. Supplementing with L-glutamine, L-glycine, and NAC can help your body get enough of those key amino acids. You could also supplement with a few grams of the branch chain amino acids (BCAAs).

B. Maintain TNF-α and hydrogen sulfide inhibition:

If possible, stay on Wellbutrin and a lower dose of Mesalamine. Mesalamine can be gradually reduced in this stage.

C. Supplementation:

- Bovine Colostrum: 5-10 grams daily during this phase, with a powder form such as that from Symbiotics being the easiest and most cost effective way of doing this.
- Phosphatidylcholine: 1 gram daily
- Increase glutathione levels with enteric-coated glutathione, or n-Acetyl l-cysteine (NAC, doesn't have to be enteric coated). NOW makes an NAC supplement that contains the selenium and molybdenum necessary for making the enzyme to turn NAC into glutathione.
- GI Revive: contains mucin (among other things) to help replenish the low levels of mucin found in people with IBD.
- Glutamine: 15 grams daily
- Selenium
- Vitamin D, Riboflavin (B2)

D. Avoid NSAIDs

Non-steriodal anti-inflammatory drugs (NSAIDs) damage the gut wall and are often purchased over the counter and consumed like candy in most Western societies. Commonly used NSAIDs include aspirin (eg Dispirin), ibuprofen (eg Nurofen), naproxen (Naprosyn), diclonfenach (eg Voltaren) and celecoxib (eg Celebrex). These are extremely bad for our gut. In fact, tests done on rats to assess the effectiveness of various colitis treatments use a high dose NSAID to initiate the onset of colitis in the rats. The thickening additive carrageenan (added to some processed foods, especially some milk substitutes) is also used to trigger colitis in rats and should similarly be avoided.

E. Lifestyle factors

Part of healing from Ulcerative Colitis is changing the way you live, permanently. A variety of lifestyle factors contribute to breakdown of the epithelial barrier, including emotional stress, alcohol, disruption of the circadian rhythm, excessive high intensity exercise and bacterial dysbiosis induced by antibiotics. Know your triggers and avoid them.

F. Microbiota rebalancing:

Microbiota rebalancing can be achieved with probiotics, fermented foods and diet. In non-responsive cases, fecal microbial transplant is an option. A diet high in fiber, resistant starches and fermented foods will help repopulate beneficial bacteria and increase SCFA production. Fermented foods such as sauerkraut are particularly handy as they add both fiber and probiotics to the diet. Nearly all vegetables can be home-fermented for a ready supply in the refrigerator at all times. Alternately fermented foods can be purchased at quality health food stores.

In addition to the probiotics mentioned in Phase 1, Bifidobacterium Longum and Brevis, and Lactobacillus Casei and Reuteri have been found to be beneficial and can been added in Phase 2. Natural Factors Ultimate Probiotic contains the first three of those, and is enteric coated. Digestive Advantage (Bacillus Coagulans BC30) and Clostridium Butyricum Miyairi are extremely valuable, as they both help boost the levels of beneficial anaerobic bacteria that can't be taken directly.

G. Re-test Intestinal Permeability:

If you have the funds, it is useful to measure your intestinal permeability/leaky gut at this point. These tests are not yet available through mainstream medical practitioners but can be ordered through a number of online labs. Once the function of your gut wall has normalized, it is time to move to Phase 3.

Phase 3—Maintain the Gut Wall

The goal of Phase 3 is to keep you in remission, while allowing you to have as normal a life as possible. There is no set timeframe for progression to this final phase. By Phase 3, you know your triggers better than anyone. Listen to your body. If possible assess your progress via an intestinal permeability test.

As discussed earlier, Inflammatory Bowel Disease arises from a hyperactive immune response to the translocation of bacteria across the epithelial barrier of the gut wall. So, if the barrier can be maintained, preventing (or at least greatly limiting) bacterial translocation, IBD should not occur. A small amount of immune modulation (with natural supplements as much as possible) will continue to be valuable though, to help handle transient leakiness due to the unavoidable situations life presents us.

Phase 3 is a preventative, modified version of Phase 2. Most of the supplements that are effective at rebuilding the gut wall have also been shown to be effective at helping to maintain it, at lower doses. Protein can be increased gradually but it is still important to minimize the other foods listed above that have been shown to cause damage to the epithelial barrier, while adopting the dietary factors (outlined in Phase 2) that have been shown to help maintain and repair the barrier.

Grains, seeds and nuts can be introduced to the diet, provided they are activated or combined with a lectin binder such as N-Acetyl L-Glucosamine. A few products are available that contain a variety of lectin binders: "Lectin Lock", Lectin Control Formula", and "GI Revive". Consumption of lectins can be limited by using sprouted grains or fermenting dough, soaking and thoroughly cooking legumes. Taking lectin binders when lectins are consumed will reduce damage to our epithelial barrier by lectins.

A very important point: after you have been healthy for a while, it is easy to become complacent. It is easy to start slacking on supplements, and get loose on the diet, and think that occasionally using

NSAIDs for a muscle pain or headache will be ok. That is a path that can lead back to misery though. If you are still unhealthy while reading this, write a note to the future, healthy you, telling yourself to NEVER get lax. You don't want to end up there again. The dietary restrictions of this protocol are nowhere near as severe as more commonly known diets (SCD, GAPS, FODMAPS, paleo, etc.). There are a lot of supplements to take. You may have a bad headache and think "what could one or two ibuprofen really do?". It can initiate damage to your gut wall, allowing bacteria to pass through, initiating the inflammatory cascade that can bring you right back to a full-blown flare. So, DON'T DO IT!

Notes on *Restore*

D r. Zachary Bush and a team of scientists from the University of Virginia (see below) have developed a product to help heal leaky gut. Based on my own positive personal experience with the product, I am including information about it here. After going on a gluten free diet, while I had a great deal of reduction in the diarrhea that accompanied my gluten intolerance, I still had problems. The product called Restore was immediately helpful and within 24 hours gave me the first formed stool I had had in four years.

Zachary Bush, MD, graduated from the University of Colorado Health Sciences Center and later became Chief Resident for the department of Internal Medicine at the University of Virginia. He is in private practice in Charlottesville VA.

David Roberts, holds a Master's Degree in public health from the Johns Hopkins School of Public Health with a focus in HIV/AIDS and international health, a Master's in biomedical engineering from the University of Virginia and Bachelor's in electrical and biomedical engineering from Duke University.

John Gildea, PhD is an Associate Professor at the University of Virginia, and the research director at the Felder Core Laboratory. About this product, Dr. Bush says:

> *"We use Restore as a foundation of health for a broad spectrum of patients. Restore does not treat any disease. Instead, it promotes strong membrane integrity through its direct and indirect effects on the tight junctions of the bowel wall and vascular systems of the body, and restoration of the bowel ecology with the unique bacterial communication attribute of the supplement. Microbiome balance and tight junction integrity are widely recognized to constitute a major portion of the human immune system, and directly affect DNA transcription of human cells to promote optimal health. Restore ingredients for gut health are comprised of purified water, a soil-based mineral supplement, Terrahydrite (TM) (Stabilized Lignite Extract), trace soil amino acids and minerals and deionized reverse osmosis water."*

If you believe you might have leaky gut, try making the lifestyle changes recommended above as well as adding probiotics to your diet and try Restore to see if it makes a difference.

References

1   12-15.5 gr hemoglobin per deciliter (dL) of blood

2   Yu-Jie Zhang, Sha Li,Ren-You Gan, Tong Zhou, et al, **Impacts of Gut Bacteria on Human Health and Diseases.** *International Journal of Molecular Science,* 2015 Apr; 16(4): 7493–7519. Published online 2015 Apr 2. doi: 10.3390/ijms16047493, PMCID: PMC4425030.

3   Eiseman B, Silen W, Bascom GS, et al., **Fecal enema as an adjunct in the treatment of pseudomembranous enterocolitis.** *Surgery.* 44 (5): 854–859. (1958), PMID 13592638.

4   Els van Nood, M.D., Josbert J. Keller, M.D., Ph.D., et al., **Duodenal Infusion of Donor Feces for Recurrent Clostridium difficile,** *New England Journal of Medicine,* 2013, 368:407-415, DOI: 10.1056/ NEJMoa1205037.

5   Center for Disease Control, https://www.cdc.gov/media/releases/2015/ p0225-clostridium-difficile.html.

6   Thomas J. Borody, Sudarshan Paramsothy, and Gaurav Agrawal, **Microbiota Transplantation: Indications, Methods, Evidence, and Future Directions,** *Current Gastroenterology Reports,* 2013; 15(8): 337. Published online 2013 Jul 14. doi: 10.1007/s11894-013-0337-1PMCID: PMC3742951.

7   Meng-Que Xu, Hai-Long Cao, Wei-Qiang Wang,et al., **Fecal microbiota transplantation broadening its application beyond intestinal disorders,** *World Journal of Gastroenterology,* 2015 Jan 7; 21(1): 102–111. Published online 2015 Jan 7. doi: 10.3748/wjg.v21.i1.102, PMCID: PMC4284325.

8   Ochman, Howard, et al, **Lateral Gene Transfer and the Nature of Bacterial Innovation,** *Nature* 405, 299-304 (18 May 2000) |

doi:10.1038/35012500, http://www.molecularalzheimer.org/files/ Ochman2000_Lateral_transfer_bacterial_DNA.PDF.

9   Willerslev, Eske, **World's Oldest Living bacteria found in Permafrost,** University of Copenhagen, *Science Daily,* August 28, 2007, A research team has for the first time ever discovered DNA from living bacteria that are more than half a million years old.

10   Coghlan, Andy, **'Resurrection bug' revived after 120,000 years,** *New Scientist,* June, 2009, https://www.newscientist.com/article/ dn17305-resurrection-bug-revived-after-120000-years.

11   Coghlan, Andy, **Resurrection Bug Revived After 120,000 Years,** *New Scientist,* https://www.newscientist.com/article/dn17305-resurrectio n-bug-revived-after-120000-years/Aguilar, Eva.

12   Aguilar, Eva, **Bacteria Make light Work of Detecting Landmines,** *Science and Development Network,* Nov 30, 2009, www.scidev.net/global/ health/.../bacteria-make-light-work-of-detecting-landmines.ht.

13   Sender, Ron, **Revised Estimates for the Number of Human and Bacteria Cells in the Body,** *PLoS Biology.* 2016 Aug; 14(8): e1002533, PMCID: PMC4991899, Published online 2016 Aug 19. doi:, 10.1371/jour-nal.pbio.1002533, and https://www.ncbi.nlm.nih.gov/pubmed/27541692, "Our analysis also updates the widely-cited 10:1 ratio, showing that the number of bacteria in the body is actually of the same order as the number of human cells, and their total mass is about 0.2 kg."

14   Van Beurden, Yvette H., et al, **Complications and long term-follow-up of fecal microbiota transplantation for treatment of recurrent Clostridium difficile infection,** Oral presentation, April, 2016, *26th European Congress of Clinical Microbiology and Infectious Diseases* (ECCMID 2016), https://www.escmid.org/escmid_publications/ escmid_elibrary/?q=fecal+transplants&id=2173&L=0&x=9&y=15.

15   Wand, Sinan, et al., **Systematic Review: Adverse Effects of Fecal Microbiota Transplantation,** *PLOS ONE,* 2016, 1(8) e0160074. Published online 2016 Aug 16, doi: 10.1371/journal pone 0161174 PMCID: PMC4986962.

16   Kelly, C.R., et al., **Fecal Microbiota Transplant for Treatment of Clostridium difficile Infection in Immunocompromised Patients,** *The American Journal of Gastroenterology,* 2014; 109 (7): 1065 DOI: 10.1038/ajg.2014.133.

17   Osman, Majid, MD MPH**, Safety and efficacy of fecal microbiota transplantation for recurrent Clostridium difficile infection from an international public stool bank: Results from a 2,050**

patient multi-center cohort, Poster Abstract: Clostridium difficile: Therapeutics, *Infectious Disease Week*, Saturday, October 29, 2016.

18   Stein, Rob, **Gut Bacteria Might Guide the Workings of Our Minds,** *National Public Radio,* November 13, 2013, https://www.npr.org/sections/health-shots/2013/11/18/244526773/gut-bacteria-might-guide-the-workings-of-our-minds.

19   Adam Hadhazy, **Think Twice: How the Gut's "Second Brain Influences Mood and Well Being,** *Scientific American*, February 12, 2010.

20   Lydiard, R. Bruce Ph.D., et al., **Prevalence of Psychiatric Disorders in Patients with Irritable Bowel Syndrome** and **The Role of Anxiety and Depression in the Irritable Bowel Syndrome,** *Behavior Research and Therapy,* Volume 28, Issue 5, 1990, Pages 401–405.

21   Peter Andrey Smith, **The tantalizing links between gut microbes and the brain,** *Nature,* 14 October 2015.

22   Hsaio, E., et al., **Indigenous Bacteria from the Gut Microbiota Regulate Host Serotonin Biosynthesis.,** *Cell*, April 9, 2015.

23   Rao, A.Venket, et al, **A randomized double-blind, placebo controlled pilot study of a probiotic in emotional symptoms of chronic fatigue syndrome,** *Gut Pathogens*, March 2009.

24   Ruixue Huang, Ke Wang, and Jianan Hu, **Effect of Probiotics on Depression: A Systematic Review and Meta-Analysis of Randomized Controlled Trials,** *Nutrients.* 2016 Aug; 8, 483. Published online 2016 Aug 6. doi: 10.3390/nu8080483 http://www.mdpi.com/2072-6643/8/8/483/htm.

25   Pritchard, Colin, Rosenorn-Lanng, Emily et al., **Deaths from Neurological Disease in the United States by sex as compared with 20 Western countries 1989–2010: Cause for concern,** P, 4 , *Surgical Neurology International*, 2015; 6: 123. Published online 2015.

26   *National institute of Mental Health*, **Mental Illness Statistics**, 2016, https://www.nimh.nih.gov/health/statistics/mental-illness.shtml.

27   Barnevik-Olsson M, Gillberg C, Fernell E., **Prevalence of autism in children of Somali origin living in Stockholm: brief report of an at-risk population.,** *Developmental Medicine and Child Neurology,* 2010 Dec;52(12):1167-8. doi: 10.1111/j.1469-8749.2010.03812.x. Epub 2010 Oct 21.

28   Becerra, Tracy, **Autism Spectrum Disorders and Race, Ethnicity, and Nativity: A Population-Based Study,** *Journal of Pediatrics,* June 2014.

29   Adams, J.B, **et al., Nutritional and metabolic status of children with autism vs. neurotypical children, and the association with autism severity,** *Nutritional Metabolism,* 2011 Jun 8;8(1):34. doi: 10.1186/1743-7075-8-34.

30   Wakefield, Andrew, et al., **The Gut-brain Axis in Childhood Developmental Disorders,** *Journal of Pediatric Gastroenterology & Nutrition,* May/June 2002, Vol 34, Issue, pp s14-s17.

31   Sharp, William G. PhD, et al., **A Systematic Review and Meta-Analysis of Intensive Multidisciplinary Intervention for Pediatric Feeding Disorders: How Standard Is the Standard of Care?** *Journal of Pediatrics,* http://dx.doi.org/10.1016/j.jpeds.2016.10.002.

32   Finegold SM, Molitoris D, Song Y, Liu C, Vaisanen ML, Bolte E, Sandler R, et al., **Gastrointestinal microflora studies in late-onset autism.,** *Clinical Infectious Disease.* 2002, Sep 1; 35, S6-S16.

33   Finegold, Sydney, Md., et al., **Short-term benefit from oral vancomycin treatment of regressive autism-,** Child Neurology- 2000, Jul;15(7):429-35, http://www.ncbi.nlm.nih.gov/pubmed/10921511-.

34   https://patents.justia.com/inventor/sydney-m-finegold.

35   Finegold, Sydney, MD., **Gastrointestinal microflora studies in late-onset autism,** *Clinical Infectious Disease,* 2002 Sep 1;35(Suppl 1):S6-S16.

36   Arnold, Carrie, **The Families that Launch their own Autism Studies,** *The Atlantic,* Sep 30, 2016, http://www.theatlantic.com/health/archive/2016/09/the-families-that-launch-their-own-autism-studies/502025/.

37   Knivsber AM1, Reichelt KL, Nødland M., **Reports on dietary intervention in autistic disorders,** *Nutritional Neuroscience,* 2001;4(1):25-37., Center for Reading Research, Stavanger College, Norway. ann-mari. knivsberg@slf.his.no.

38   Reichelt KL, Knivsberg AM, **The possibility and probability of a gut-to-brain connection in autism,** *Ann Clin Psychiatry.* 2009 Oct-Dec;21(4):205-11.

39   Shelly A. Buffington, et al, **Microbial Reconstitution Reverses Maternal Diet-Induced Social and Synaptic Deficits in Offspring,** *Cell* 165, 1762-1775, June 16, 2016, DOI: http://dx.doi.org/10.1016/j.cell.2016.06.001.

40   Elaine Y. Hsiao, et al, **Microbiota Modulate Behavioral and Physiological Abnormalities Associated with Neurodevelopmental Disorders,** *Cell,* Volume 155, Issue 7, 19 December 2013, Pages 1451–1463.

41 Mayer E, **Altered Brain-Gut Axis in Autism: Comorbidity or Causative Mechanisms?** *Journal Gastroenterology,* 2014, https://www.ncbi.nlm.nih.gov/pubmed/25145752.

42 Mazmanian, Sarkis, Hsaio, Elaine, et al, **Microbiota Modulates Gut Physiology and Behavorial Abnormalities Associated with Autism,** *Cell,* December 2013).

43 Perlmutter, David, M.D., ***Brain Maker,*** 2015, Little & Brown, p. 126,127.

44 Kang Dae-Wook, Adams, James B., Gregory, Ann, C., Borody, Thomas, Fasano, Alessio, et al., **Microbiota Transfer Therapy alters gut ecosystem and improves gastrointestinal and autism symptoms: an open-label study (18 patients),** *Microbiome,* Jan 23, 2017, 5:10, https://doi.org/10.1186/s40168-016-0225-7.

45 Ward, Linda, et al., **Combined oral fecal capsules plus fecal enema as treatment of late onset autism spectrum disorder in children: report of a small case series,** University of Calgary and Alberta Health Services, Calgary, Canada, *Open Forum Infectious Diseases*, Volume 3, Issue suppl_1, 25, October 2016, 1 December 2016, 2219, https://doi.org/10.1093/ofid/ofw172.1767.

46 Li, Qinrui, Han, Ying, Belle, Angel, Hagerman, Randi J., **The Gut Microbiota and Autism Spectrum Disorders,** *Frontiers in Cellular Neuroscience*, 28 April 2017 | https://doi.org/10.3389/fncel.2017.00120).

47 Rowan, Karen, **Inflammatory Bowel Disease on Rise in US,** *CDC Weekly Morbidity and Mortality Report,* November 4, 2016 06:29pm ET.

48 Ghosh, Subatra, et al, **Inflammatory Bowel Disease: A Global Disease,** *Saudi J Gastroenterology.* 2013 Jan-Feb; 19(1): 1–2.doi: 10.4103/1319-3767.105905.

49 Crohn's and Colitis Foundation of America, http://www.crohnscolitisfoundation.org.

50 Crohn's and Colitis Foundation of America, http://www.crohnscolitisfoundation.org.

51 Colman RJ, et al, **Fecal microbiota transplantation as therapy for inflammatory bowel disease: a systematic review and meta-analysis,** *J Crohn's Colitis.* 2014 Dec 1; 8(12): 1569–1581. Published online 2014 Sep 13. doi: 10.1016/j.crohns.2014.08.006.

52 Dong Y1, Huang W1, Zhu D1, Mao H2, Su P2, **Fecal Microbiota Transplantation for Ulcerative Colitis: A Systematic Review and Meta-Analysis.** Shi Y, *PLoS One*, 2016 Jun 13;11(6): e0157259. doi: 10.1371/journal.pone.0157259.

53 Paramsothy, S., et al., **Multi-donor intense faecal microbiota transplantation is an effective treatment for resistant ulcerative**

colitis: a randomized placebo-controlled trial, European Crohn's and Colitis Organization, *Abstracts &Oral presentations 2016*, OP017 S.Paramsothy, et al.

54   Rubio-Tapia, A1, et al., **Increased prevalence and mortality in undiagnosed celiac disease,** *Gastroenterology.* 2009 Jul;137(1):88-93. doi: 10.1053/j.gastro.2009.03.059. Epub 2009 Apr 10.

55   Elliott, Roger, personal testimony, report in its entirety at: http://www. celiactravel.com/blog/fmt-treatment-at-the-uk-taymount-clinic/.

56   Samsel, Anthony, et al., **Glyphosate, pathways to modern diseases II: Celiac sprue and gluten intolerance,** *Interdisciplinary Toxicology*, Volume 6, Issue 4 (Dec 2013), p. 159-164.

57   Capel, Paul, Environmental Chemist and Head of the agricultural chemicals team at the U.S. Geological Survey Office, U.S. Department of the interior. A study from the U.S. Geological Survey, accepted for publication online ahead of print in the journal *Environmental Toxicology and Chemistry*, titled, **Pesticides in Mississippi air and rain: A comparison between 1995 and 2007,** (Roundup herbicide (aka glyphosate) and its still-toxic degradation byproduct aminomethylphosphonic acid, or AMPA, were found in over 75% of the air and rain samples tested from Mississippi in 2007.)

58   Samsel, Anthony, Senefee, Stephanie, **Glyphosate, pathways to modern diseases II: Celiac sprue and gluten intolerance,** *Interdisciplinary Toxicology*, **Published Online**: 2014-03- 11, DOI: https://doi.org/10.2478/intox-20, 13-0026, December 4, 2013, Vol 6, issue 4.

59   Fasano, A., et al., **Leaky Gut and Autoimmune Disease,** *Clin Rev Allergy Immunol.,* 2012 Feb;42(1):71-8. doi: 10.1007/s12016-011-8291-x.

60   Wahls, Terry, *The Wahls Protocol,* Avery, 2014, p. 96-97.

61   Blum, Susan, MD, *Immune System Recovery Plan*, Scribner, 2013, p. 186-190.

62   Fasano, A., et al., **Zonulin and Its Regulation of Intestinal Barrier Function: The Biological Door to Inflammation, Autoimmunity, and Cancer,** *Physiological Reviews*, Published 1 January 2011 Vol. 91 no. 1, 151-175 DOI: 10.1152/physrev.00003.2008.

63   Chutkan, Robynnne K., *Could Leaky Gut Be What's Troubling You?* (Dr. Chutkan, Professor of Medicine, Georgetown University Hospital, Founder and Medical Director of the Digestive Center for Women) Posted on 2/20/2013, Dr. Oz website.

64 Mangiola, Francesca, et al. **Gut microbiota in autism and mood disorders,** *World J Gastroenterol,* 2016 Jan 7; 22(1): 361–368, Published online 2016 Jan 7. doi: 10.3748/wjg.v22.i1.361,PMCID: PMC4698498.

65 Nakazawa, Donna J., **The Autoimmune Epidemic,** Touchstone Publishing, 2008, Forward by Douglas Kerr, M.D., Ph.D.

66 Campbell, Andrew W., **Autoimmunity and the Gut,** *Autoimmune Disease,* 2014; 2014: 152428. Published online 2014 May 13. doi: 10.1155/2014/152428, PMCID: PMC4036413.

67 Campbell, Andrew W., **Autoimmunity and the Gut,** *Autoimmune Disease,* 2014; 2014: 152428. Published online 2014 May 13. doi: 10.1155/2014/152428, PMCID: PMC4036413.

68 Fields, Helen, **The Gut: Where Bacteria and Immune System Meet,** *Hopkins Medicine,* https://www.hopkinsmedicine.org/research/advancements-in-research/fundamentals/in-depth/the-gut-where-bacteria-and-immune-system-meet, November 2015.

69 Filiano, Anthony J., **What Does Immunology Have to do With Brain Development and Neuropsychiatric Disorders? Interactions of innate and adaptive immunity in brain development and function,** *Brain Research,* Volume 1617, 18 August 2015, Pages 18–27.

70 Mazmanian, Sarkis, K., et al., **The gut microbiome shapes intestinal immune responses during health and disease,** *National Review Immunology,* 2009 May; 9(5): 313–323, doi: 10.1038/nri2515, PMCID: PMC4095778, NIHMSID: NIHMS525429.

71 Purchiaroni, F, et al., **Cross Talk, The role of intestinal microbiota and the immune system,** *European Review Medical Pharmacology Science,* 2013 Feb;17(3):323-33.

72 Meng-Que Xu, et al, **Fecal microbiota transplantation broadening its application beyond intestinal disorders,** *World J Gastroenterol.* 2015 Jan 7; 21(1): 102–111, Published online 2015 Jan 7. doi: 10.3748/wjg.v21.i1.102, PMCID: PMC4284325.

73 The National Multiple Sclerosis Society Website: https://www.nationalmssociety.org/What-is-MS

74 Rumah, Kareem Rashid, Et al., **Isolation of Clostridium perfringens Type B in an Individual at First Clinical Presentation of Multiple Sclerosis Provides Clues for Environmental Triggers of the Disease.** *PLoS ONE,* 2013; 8 (10): e76359 DOI: 10.1371/journal.pone.0076359.

75 Mazmanian SK1, Liu CH, Tzianabos AO, Kasper DL., **An immunomodulatory molecule of symbiotic bacteria directs maturation of the host immune system.,** *Cell.* 2005;122:107–118.

76   Borody, T.J., Leis. S.M., **Fecal Microbiota Transplantation in M.S.,** August 25, 2012, online at fecalmicrobiotatransplant.com. and Borody TJ, et al, **Fecal microbiota transplantation (FMT) in multiple sclerosis** (MS), *Am J Gastroenterol.* 2011;106: S352.

77   Jacob, Aglaee, MS, RD, **Gut Health and Autoimmune Disease, Research Suggests Digestive Abnormalities May Be the Underlying Cause,** *Today's Dietitian*, **Vol. 15 No. 2 P. 38. February 2013,** http://www.todaysdietitian.com/newarchives/021313p38.shtml.

78   Vaahtovuo J, Munukka E, Korkeamaki M, Luukkainen R, Toivanen P., **Fecal microbiota in early rheumatoid arthritis.** *J Rheumatol.* Aug 2008;35(8):1500-1505.

79   Olena, Abbey, **Microbes May Impact Autoimmunity,** *The Scientist*, November 6, 2013, http://www.the- scientist.com/?articles.view/articleNo/38206/title/Gut-Microbes-May-Impact-Autoimmunity/.

80   Sampson, Timothy, R., **Gut Microbiota Regulate Motor Deficits and Neuroinflammation in a Model of Parkinson's Disease,** *Cell,* Volume 167, Issue 6, p1469–1480.e12, 1 December 2016.

81   Frémont M, Coomans D, Massart S, De Meirleir K. **High-throughput 16S rRNA gene sequencing reveals alterations of intestinal micro-biota in myalgic encephalomyelitis/chronic fatigue syndrome,** *Anaerobe*, 2013 Aug;22:50-6. doi: 10.1016/j.anaerobe.2013.06.002. Epub 2013 Jun 19.

82   Borody TJ, Nowak A, Finlayson S. **The GI microbiome and its role in chronic fatigue syndrome: A summary of bacterio-therapy.** *Australasian College of Nutritional and Environmental Medicine,* 2012;31:3.

83   Olszak, T. *et al.* **Microbial exposure during early life has persistent effects on natural killer T cell function,** *Science*, http://dx.doi.org/10.1126/science.1219328, 2012.

84   Hullar, Meredith, A.J, et al., **Gut Microbes, Diet, and Cancer,** *Cancer Treat Research*, 2015 Jan 1., Published in final edited form as: Cancer Treat Res. 2014; 159: 377–399., doi: 10.1007/978-3-642-380075_22, PMCID: PMC4121395, NIHMSID: NIHMS578625).

85   Gopalakrishnan, V., Wargo, J, et al., **Response to anti-PD-1 based therapy in metastatic melanoma patients is associated with the diversity and composition of the gut microbiome**, *Cancer Research*, July 2017, DOI: 10.1158/1538-7445.AM2017-2672.

86   University of Texas Cancer Center, **Gut bacteria associated with cancer immunotherapy response in melanoma,** *ScienceDaily,*

https://www.sciencedaily.com/releases/2017/02/170221222752.htm, 21 Feb 2017.

87   Routy, Bernard, et al, **Gut microbiome influences efficacy of PD-1– based immunotherapy against epithelial tumors,** *Science*, 02 Nov 2017: eaan3706, DOI: 10.1126/science.aan,3706)

88   Cheema, A.K., Schiestl,Robert H., **Chemopreventive Metabolites Are Correlated with a Change in Intestinal Microbiota Measured in A-T Mice and Decreased Carcinogenesis.** *PLoS ONE*, 2016 DOI: 10.1371/journal.pone.0151190.

89   Dethlefsen L, Huse S, Sogin ML, Relman DA, **The Pervasive Effects of an Antibiotic on the Human Gut Microbiota,** *Journal PLoS Biology*, 2008, http://journals.plos.org/plosbiology/article?id=10.1371/journal.pbio.0060280.

90   Kaplan, Gilaad, G. , MD, MPH,et al, **The Inflammatory Bowel Diseases and Ambient Air Pollution: A Novel Association,** *American Journal of Gastroenterology*, 2010 Nov; 105(11): 2412–2419, Published online 2010 Jun 29. doi: 10.1038/ajg.2010.252.

91   Kaplan, Gilaad, G. , MD, MPH,et al, **The Inflammatory Bowel Diseases and Ambient Air Pollution: A Novel Association,** *American Journal of Gastroenterology,* 2010 Nov; 105(11): 2412–2419, Published online 2010 Jun 29. doi: 10.1038/ajg.2010.252.

92   Salim, Saad Y, et al, **Air pollution effects on the gut microbiota, a link between exposure and inflammatory disease,** *Gut Microbes.* 2014 Mar 1; 5(2): 215–219, Published online 2013 Dec 20. doi: 10.4161/gmic.27251.

93   Benedict C, et al, **Gut Microbiota and Glucometabolic Alterations in Response to Recurrent Partial Sleep Deprivation in Normal-weight Young Individuals**, *Molecular Metabolism*, 2016, in press. DOI: 10.1016/j.molmet.2016.10.003.

94   Clarke, S, Murphy, E., **Exercise and associated dietary extremes impact on gut microbial diversity,** *Gut* 2014; 63 1838-1839 Published Online First: 09 Jun 2014. doi: 10.1136/gutjnl-2014-307305.

95   Chutkan, Robin MD, ***The Microbiome Solution,*** Penguin Random House, LLC., 2015.

96   Anthony, A, **I had the bacteria in my gut analyzed. And this may be the future of medicine**, *The Guardian,* February 2014, https://www.theguardian.com/science/2014/feb/11/gut-biology-health-bacteria-future-medicine.

97   Anthony, A, **I had the bacteria in my gut analyzed. And this may be the future of medicine**, *The Guardian,* February 2014, https://

www.theguardian.com/science/2014/feb/11/gut-biology-health-bacteri
a-future-medicine.

98   Moayyedi P, Et al., **Fecal Microbiota Transplantation Induces
      Remission in Patients With Active Ulcerative Colitis in
      a Randomized Controlled Trial,** *Gastroenterology,* 2015
      Jul;149(1):102-109.e6. doi: 10.1053/j.gastro.2015.04.001.

99   Shi, Yanqiang, et al, **Fecal Microbiota Transplantation for Ulcerative
      Colitis: A Systematic Review and Meta-Analysis,** *PLoS One,* 2016;
      11(6): e0157259. Published online 2016 Jun 13. doi: 10.1371/journal.
      pone.0157259.

100   Paramsothy, S, et al. **Multidonor intensive faecal microbiota
      transplantation for active ulcerative colitis: A randomised
      placebo-controlled trial.** *Lancet* 2017 Feb 14; *[e-pub].* (http://dx.doi.
      org/10.1016/S0140-6736(17)30182-4.

101   Siegmund, B. **Is intensity the solution for FMT in ulcerative
      colitis?** *Lancet* 2017 Feb 14; *[e-pub].* (http://dx.doi.org/10.1016/
      S0140-6736(17)30313-6.

102   *The Fecal Transplant Foundation,* thefecaltransplantfoundation.org/

Printed in Great Britain
by Amazon